CATAWAMPUS

The Fertility Process from a Man's Perspective

STUART A. BURKHALTER

HUGENSLOP
PRESS

NASHVILLE, TENNESSEE

Hugenslop Press

Nashville, Tennessee

www.stuartburkhalter.com

Book design by Diana Wade

First Edition: April 2014

Disclaimers: Every effort has been made to accurately present the views and activities presented herein. The publisher and author regret any unintentional inaccuracies or omissions and do not assume responsibility for the opinions gathered for this book. Neither the publisher nor the author of the information presented herein shall be liable for any loss of profit or any other commercial damages, including but not limited to special, incidental, consequential, or other damages.

For Julie

Cambodian Jungle

"Do you even want to have a baby?"

My friend Newt called me at work one day not long after the first IVF transfer had failed. Newt had made it a habit to call me periodically at work so that I would hear the crack of our receptionist buzzing over the intercom that there was a "Newt" for me on Line X. He never called for the purpose of discussing fertility concerns, and in fact, Newt was not aware, as far as I knew, of what IVF was, or that we had recently undergone a transfer, or that we had undergone any fertility treatments whatsoever. Instead, he appeared to enjoy periodic work phone conversations with an old high school friend.

When he called this time around March 2012, I was finally looking to tell someone something—to talk to someone other than my wife—and thus, when he asked how things were going, I told him honestly.

"You know, Newt, not so great."

I work in an old, stone house on West End Avenue in Nashville. Apparently, in the eighteen-hundreds, stately homes like this with multiple chimneys, drawing rooms, and dark wood covering all available surfaces, used to line this primary thoroughfare leading up from downtown and the Cumberland River west into the suburbs. Now our building is sandwiched between a Pizza Hut Express on one side and what was a Mrs. Winner's, then a Church's Chicken, then a shuttered Church's Chicken, and now an AT&T store on the other.

About twenty years ago, before my law firm moved in, an architecture firm bought the house, left the original structure essentially intact, and built an extension of office space on the back. The extension was cutting-edge and modern for its time: spiral staircases, exposed pipes, skylights, and an entire wall of windows facing west. My office is on the lowest floor, below street level, and my view out my office door through this window wall is an alley and, beyond that, the faded, beige-yellow brick of Pizza Hut. The pizza employees periodically drag out various cooking utensils and trays and spray them down with a hose in the alley. At other times, a crazy man may shuffle through.

Despite the limits of this view, I tend to avoid shutting my office door if at all possible, because otherwise, I might feel like I'm buried underground with only piles of paper to keep me company. But, on this particular occasion, I got up and sealed myself in.

I told Newt about our experience through the fertility process thus far, and in particular, the feeling of living in constant, all-consuming frustration—a frustration that had recently bottomed out, with a whimper, after a failed IVF transfer in Dallas.

In the midst of my extended confession, he interrupted, "I don't know if this is even an appropriate question at this point, but, I mean, do you even want to have a baby?"

I laughed and said that conversation—or at least, that particular topic— was half-heartedly raised (by me) and quickly dropped long, long ago. So long ago, in fact, that remembering back to the time where *that* was a concern of mine seemed about as removed from the present as a horse-drawn carriage might, clopping through the alley outside my office, while blue chimney smoke silently billowed overheard.

Did I even want to have a baby? Prior to any and all trying and failing? Prior to the fertility treatments? I have no idea. Sure. Always thought I would. I probably thought it was going to be a major change that I didn't quite want to delve into just yet. I probably thought that having a life centered around baby showers and baby photos and love for babies was beneath me. I probably thought babies and children, in general, were a bit more obnoxious than they were cute. But now, I didn't care whether I "wanted to" then or not. What I did know was that I wanted, desperately wanted, and ached for whatever we were currently doing to be successful and complete and over.

My wife, Julie, however, was different. She said then and she'd say confidently now, without hesitation, that she had always dreamed of being a mother. That it was always of primary importance. I had known this, of course, but I also knew that there were other factors to consider.

Julie and I both graduated from the University of Virginia in 2003. We spent the next two years or so in Washington, D.C. She worked for a trade association. I bombed job interviews.[1] I eventually got a glorified administrative position at a local D.C. government agency. I spent the first six months reading the *Washington Post* at work and lamenting the state of my professional existence and the last six months working on a movie with my old high school friend Charlie.

After shooting the movie—a thirty-two minute short film—in early 2005, Julie and I moved to New York City. She got a job as a buyer for a major women's clothing retailer. I worked with Charlie to finish up the movie and found part-time work watching television at a market research company. Later, I was a paralegal. The movie ran its course.[2] Eventually, a switch flipped in my professional decision-making and I decided to go to law school. In 2007 Julie and I moved from New York City, got married in Charlottesville, and, after the honeymoon, drove to Nashville, my hometown. I started law school the next day at Vanderbilt. Julie found work about three months later as a buyer for a major men's shoe retailer, based in Nashville.

Baby discussions certainly arose during the three years of law school, but Julie didn't push it. It was theoretically not the right time. At first, the topic was wildly alien to me. But, then, like anything else, it began to make more sense—or else, all of my rational excuses ceased to be rational—and, at some point, it was decided: Let's wait until after law school. Then everything would be ready.

Therefore, we did not actively start trying to get pregnant until after I graduated from law school and, actually, until after the Tennessee bar exam in July 2010. That we delayed "trying" not only until law school was over but until *the bar exam* was over three months later seems laughable to me now. I don't know if I anticipated a baby spontaneously emerging and taking a few glances around the room after sweet, unprotected love-making or that unprotected sex would perhaps distract me from the task of memorizing flashcards of legal concepts, but back then, it seemed like another conversation—a different conversation—that I couldn't quite handle until I had completed the job at hand.

We were both twenty-nine at the time, and so perhaps this concept should not have been as foreign to me as it was, but the peer-group baby boom had not yet begun. Thus, my apparent inability to contemplate two differing

---

[1] During one, I found myself telling some poor bastard a story about a Barnes and Noble gift card—as in, I had such a gift card, and I planned on using it at some point. The end. Please hire me.

[2] A "Best Short Drama" award at the now-defunct Blue Ridge Mountain Southwest Virginia Vision Film Festival in Roanoke, Virginia, being the highlight.

aspects of life that might require my attention, simultaneously, had not been exposed just yet as short-sighted.

Julie ceased taking birth control pills one year before we started "trying." I remember her doing that and telling me that she was doing so, but even then, I did not understand why. That would just be the first of many things I did not fully intuit during this process. Instead, it was simply understood through the vibrant and brimming-with-information, female grapevine that the birth control pill should be discontinued far before actually attempting a pregnancy. So, sure, that's what we did.

At some point I heard the phrase "pulling the goalie" used as a metaphor for ceasing all birth control. But it was only after we were struggling, deep and confused along the fertility trail, that this phrase sprung up and seemed to me, like many other things at the time, highly inaccurate. I knew this particular metaphor was related to hockey, but in my mind, I always associated it with soccer. And so I thought pulling the goalie was like pulling the keeper and I was standing there waiting on an empty-net penalty kick, where probably ninety-six times out of a hundred I could manage to knock it in. Of course, I was mistaken. Instead, in the midst of our experience, it appeared to me that for this analogy to be remotely accurate I would need to be on ice, on skates for the first time since fifth grade, standing behind my own goal, maybe with a soggy mop instead of a stick.

And I wondered: Why did we even have birth control pills? Why had we been bothering with condoms every time we had face-melting sex if it was so difficult to have success when we were in there, with no restraints, letting loose to our hearts' content? In short, if I had known it was going to be this hard, I would have approached this entire process far, far differently. We wouldn't have waited this bloody long!

But an arbitrary line had been drawn: law school, bar exam, then sure, let's give it a shot. Of course, after the bar exam, with a never-ending, legal career on the immediate horizon, we planned a trip to Asia. And when taking a trip to Asia, certain government agencies recommend taking drugs for malaria, yellow fever, Japanese donkey flu, and the like. Now, when we were finally set to begin, we had a medical professional telling us that my wife shouldn't be taking this medicine if she was pregnant or trying to get pregnant.

Julie was, understandably, more than ready to get the whole process started. Right on the cusp of actually making progress, she did not want to be told that she needed to hold off a little bit longer while we were on a fourteen-day trip overseas and then, oh yeah, for a couple of weeks after we returned while the medicine gradually trickled out of her body. Before we had heard this news, we had been making jokes about the mystery and intrigue of starting to "try" in Asia—a baby conceived in Kuala Lumpur! Abdul Burkhalter! So upon hearing this, she was upset.

I had doubts that this was that pivotal of a predicament. At the same time, I understood the frustration. And likewise, I understood that my uninformed opinion that it was more than likely not a problem—the first of many times where I was asked for an uninformed medical opinion (and gave one), that fourteen days was not that terribly long of a time, and that it was highly unlikely that anything would occur in that fourteen days—there I actually was correct—did not salve her angst. She called her uncle, a doctor in Georgia, to get his advice. And before I knew it, in another sign of things to come, the entire enterprise became a semi-public one.

This is true more for women than men, but at least in our particular social circles, there seems to be a certain point in time after which women simply know that another woman is having an issue. At some particular stage, there is either a reason or a problem. Once it became readily apparent that my wife and I not only had a problem but had passed a fair number of trail markers on the unkempt, fertility trail and were rapidly, blindly, and hysterically forging deeper, Julie became, whether she wanted to or not, a resource for others. Ask Julie; she's done it all!

For me, at the beginning and through many months of this process, I was evasive and gave friends vague statements like, well, my wife is having surgery that day, so no, we can't go to dinner. It's no big deal though. It's casual surgery. I swear, it's fine. After extended darker times, though, I found telling a male friend like Newt worthwhile to, at the very least, provide me with some basic perspective. I needed a reminder of normalcy that can be lacking when you're so deep on the fertility trail that you're incapable of waking up to what are typical concerns of the world like, say, "Hey, man, do you even want to have a baby?"

Eventually, the call ended. I opened the door to my office to let a sense of the outside seep back in and returned to work.

I hung up the phone that day feeling a measure of relief. Nothing had changed, of course. We were still as clueless and wanting as before, and our journey through the fertility process was destined to continue. But I felt then, as I do now, that details of our experience needed to be remembered and that the story needed to be told to someone.

In the end, Julie's uncle said that the antimalarial medicine should not be a major concern, but if we were alarmed, she might just want to wait a little while, a week or so, or alternatively, she could stop taking the medicine earlier so that it would be out of her system sooner rather than later. I don't know if prematurely ceasing the antimalarial medicine was on her mind when we biked through the Cambodian jungle led by a fifteen-year-old Cambodian boy to crumbling stone temples, abandoned by ancient kings first and, more recently, by tourists, as these particular sights were impressively far off a tourist-trod path of any sort, with rain persistently coming down, and a steadily rising river by our side without concern for us in our twelve-cent ponchos. In the end, I imagine she was balancing those concerns—malaria, drowning in a Cambodian jungle, running over a landmine—along with any number of others, while still gliding along with a grin on her face.

And that attitude is similar to what I encountered from her on what felt like countless occasions throughout this process: Julie, trying to keep down overwhelming, legitimate worries, while always maintaining a conviction that what we were doing was necessary, that all of this had to be done in order to have ourselves a sweet little baby.

But that is how our journey began: in Cambodia, just me, my wife, and a beautiful Cambodian boy. Or else, it actually began in a Hong Kong hotel room, after quitting the malaria medicine, uncertain that the decision was the right one, uncertain if the medicine might still be in her system, basing our understanding of what to do and when to do it on one-off, medical advice. In short, in the final sign of things to come, we were unsure, anxious, harried, and full of drugs as it began.

Ninth Avenue South, Nashville, Tennessee

"Do you know what I'm wearing?
I'm wearing a tie."

While I was studying for a semester at the University of Nottingham in college, I joined Charlie and a Texan I had met in my travels, and the three of us journeyed to stay with friends in Seville, Spain, for the Feria bullfighting festival. The festival was an over-blown, fantastic carnival, and we drank many rebujitos and rode old-fashioned carnival rides and attended a bullfight and took pictures of horses wearing tassels. In general, we marauded, trying not to be drunken Americans, because we thought—or at least I thought—that we were different: significantly less base and ridiculous than the many other drunken, American college kids punching each other out outside of bars. In hindsight, I suppose doubt may exist that our particular method of partying was any more sophisticated than the rest, but at the time, high on youthful exuberance and alcohol, I felt sure we were different.

Apropos of a supreme lack of sophistication, however, was the fact that during my travels, I developed what I thought was a healthy distaste for gypsies selling flowers and, generally annoying my twenty-one-year-old self. After one long day of binge-drinking at the Feria, I found myself with prosciutto legs dangling above my head, in a large tent full of merrymaking Spanish families, and having a meaningful conversation with Charlie, who was telling me about his college friend who had recently died in a motorcycle accident. I appreciated the moment of seriousness. I felt a desire to express, not necessarily my understanding because I had not experienced anything of the sort, but at least an attempt at fellow-feeling, as I recognized the magnitude of his loss, when an older gypsy woman appeared with a flower to sell. Although

I was not angry in any way or particularly offended, I had built up so much talk about my dislike for gypsies that I thought it necessary to act on all that bluster, and, in a momentary spur, I knocked the flower out of her hand. She slapped my hand once, quickly and not overly aggressively, picked up her flower, and then moved on.

Perhaps because of bad horror movies[3] or, maybe, good Disney cartoons,[4] this memory flashed through my mind quite a few times during our fertility struggles. I obviously don't believe that I had been cursed by a disgruntled gypsy woman in Spain or, actually, that there was any rational connection between the two events. In waking life, thinking rationally and appropriately, I could recognize that it was just my anxious and bizarre mind, racing in all directions, thinking strange thoughts for no particular reason other than it could. But in the end, it was there, and such a thought had a tendency to come around now and again, perhaps while lying in bed, not yet fully engaged in the world, and wondering.[5]

***

This first, initial stretch of the fertility trail was nothing exotic, nothing we hadn't dabbled in before: sex and doctors' offices. I was, of course, woefully unaware of the long, unexpected journey that I was beginning to undertake without proper support of any kind, soon-to-be-blood-and/or-semen-stained pocket handkerchiefs[6] or otherwise. Because, even with whatever minor concerns we had at the beginning, this experience was still something that I thought would be a straightforward affair, where time and simple "patience" (by which I mean one month or two of "struggle" before everything politely took its place) would get the job done.

In the beginning, unlike many others who may have approached this problem from the more traditional position of trying and trying and trying and failing and failing and failing, our situation was a tad different. Nothing

---

[3] See *Thinner* (Paramount, 1996) (car accident); *Drag Me To Hell* (Universal, 2009) (refusal to extend mortgage loan).

[4] See *Beauty and the Beast* (Disney, 1991) (being a jerk to an old lady who shows up at your door in the middle of the night).

[5] See William Gay, *Provinces of Night* (Doubleday, 2000) ("These hours before first light were merciless. You could not go back to sleep and it was too early to get up and the things you had done or not done lay in your mind immovable as misshapen things you'd erected from stone.").

[6] See J.R.R. Tolkien, *The Hobbit* (Allen & Unwin, 1937).

too extreme, but we started actively trying from a position of more-than-typical uncertainty and doubt, because from the start, we had two tangible issues that plagued us with worry. The first of these was an irregular period.

I could tell, early on, that something was amiss. We had one, although probably more, of these bathroom conversations:

"What is it?" I asked.

"There's still nothing—this can't be right. I'm on at least Day Thirty-Seven, and there's nothing," Julie said.

I thought that it was more than likely still completely normal though, right? "Well, I'm sure it takes some time to get back to regularity."

"Yeah," she responded, "but I've been off the Pill for over a year."

"What was it like before the Pill?" I said.

"Honestly, that was so long ago, I just don't think it matters."

OK, I thought, I'm sure this isn't the first time this issue has ever come up. "Well, I mean, if there is something actually wrong—I'm sure this is probably normal—but if not, have you told your doctor about it yet?"

We were back in Nashville after our trip. I had started work. September 2010 came and went, and there was obviously no success. When the period did occur, it was more in the forty-day range. What the irregularity meant, I had no idea and, in fact, I never did receive a straight answer. Thus, even looking back now, I cannot tell you if the irregularity had anything to do with the infertility. Irregularity may have been a symptom of a problem that would inhibit fertilization or maybe it never was. It could have been something significant; it could have been nothing; it could have been diet; it could have been entirely meaningless.

Perhaps we could have dealt with the irregularity by looking past it, by accepting it as an individual idiosyncrasy that, in the end, did not necessarily mean that Julie was infertile—just irregular—which meant our opportunities might be fewer or more sporadic, but still just as good, so long as we could time it right. Unfortunately, there was more opportunity for worry to come.

After the October cycle, which was again irregular, there was a second issue: menstrual spotting that began four to seven days prior to the period's beginning. Having been off birth control for over a year, this was not the first time that this spotting had occurred, and to Julie, this was a serious concern.

First, it was, theoretically, a symptom of PCOS (Polycystic Ovarian

Syndrome).[7] PCOS was one of those ailments that you do not ever remember hearing about from anyone at any point in your life until you do, and then, suddenly, it seems terribly popular—so popular that it would seem that you happen to be living in a statistically anomalous subset of the population where luteinizing hormones had run berserk. It was commonplace in female chatter, though, where concrete answers in the form of diagnosable medical conditions were highly valued and preferable to the alternative of, "Yeah, sorry, keep trying."

Second, for whatever reason, the spotting also became a tell-tale sign that perhaps my wife was not ovulating whatsoever. I do not remember specifically how that particular conclusion whirligigged its way into our conversation, but as soon as it did, it established deep roots,[8] and was, thenceforth, a tough one to rationally overcome. Because, if you're taking shots on goal, and for whatever reason, they're going wide—that's one thing. If the goal isn't there at all, then it makes the whole thing, all the worry, thought, concern, and planning, even sillier…while time continues to tick by, day after day.

At this time, we did make halfhearted attempts to verify whether ovulation was occurring. First, my wife bought the over-the-counter, ovulation-predictor urination sticks.[9] Unfortunately, she rarely got positive ovulation results from these, which only seemed to confirm our worries. Partly, I believe, the problem was the irregularity because, of course, the sticks aren't set up for a forty-day cycle, and so we may have been missing the appropriate urination day. Otherwise, the answer was never clear; it was never a plus or minus or multiple pink lines or a giant, smiley Humpty

---

[7] If someone came swinging on a vine into my house wearing a wild donkey suit and asked me to explain what PCOS is and why it can be a cause of "infertility," I wouldn't be able to say, which is moderately ridiculous for many reasons, but primarily because PCOS acted as a bogeyman for an extended period of time in my life. Later, I did track down an impressively comprehensive and informative book that my mother-in-law had sent my wife at some point during the process. I'll give you their definition of PCOS, although, for laughs, just nouns and adjectives because that seems closer to my actual experience of being told this medical information: "hormonal disorder luteinizing hormone ovaries testosterone male hormone surge ovulation overdrive follicle-stimulating hormone pituitary gland egg follicle abnormal rhythm ovulation." Julie Vargo & Maureen Regan, *A Few Good Eggs: Two Chicks Dish on Overcoming the Insanity of Infertility*, 24 (Regan Books, 2005).

[8] See *The Lord of the Rings: The Fellowship of the Ring* (New Line, 2001) ("The trees are strong, my Lord. Their roots go deep.").

[9] These cost somewhere around $30 for the more expensive kind, but I'm not going to start running the tab on this journey just yet. We'll chalk up this particular trip to Walgreens to "living."

Dumpty with two thumbs up, mouthing the words, "This guy!" Thus, it did not provide the certainty we were looking for and was not something that we decided to invest much time or money in.

Julie also made some attempts to chart her temperature for a couple of months. This process requires the wife (again) to take her temperature at the same time every day, immediately upon waking up. The idea is that her body temperature spikes if she ovulates and stays high if she conceives, and drops if she does not. Again, this was not conclusive for us and never terribly useful. Because if she was on a forty- to fifty-day cycle, which days were most likely for ovulation? Day Twenty-Eight to Day Thirty-Three? And can you confidently take your temperature thirty times in a row, every morning, seeing nothing, with a constant fear that you might not be ovulating whatsoever, and somehow, have great confidence come Day Thirty-Two that you are giving it a legitimate shot? Or even if you start on Day Twenty or Twenty-Five, won't there always be a worry that you might have missed it? That this month of all months, for whatever incomprehensible reason, might have been the one month where everything returned to normal, and you had an average thirty-day cycle? It seemed a major time commitment for something that, at best, was a bit of peace of mind.

Needless to say, it seemed like too many problematic variables had been thrown into a process that was supposed to be all-natural and organic. We were looking for exactitude, confirmation that our tries were worthwhile and were, at least, capable of success. And vague lines on a contraption from Walgreens and temperature readings on a slapdick thermometer were providing neither certainty nor solace.

We moved quickly to those we believed would have answers.

***

At this time, we lived on Ninth Avenue South in the 12 South district in Nashville. Twelfth Avenue South was an old trolley line. If you take a hard right after West End Avenue has turned into Broadway on its way downtown and ride Twelfth for a few miles through a variety of different commercial stretches, alternately completely revamped and not, and housing projects, not revamped whatsoever, you'll reach the 12 South neighborhood. It's an "older" neighborhood, which in Nashville means it has sidewalks. Single-family homes packed in a grid of hilly streets.

We had lived there since the start of law school in an unrenovated, two-story bungalow. The neighborhood was still in the last, fading moments of its "transitioning" period and had not yet embarked on its next, current stage of being razed, remade, and booming.

**

I felt a certain amount of distance from the early medical visits as I was receiving most of the information filtered through my wife. That's not to say that hearing it from the physician was much better. I certainly experienced man's initial sense of oh-wait-just-wait-until-I-get-in-there-to-talk-to-this-doctor-I'll-get-some-straight-answers-out-of-her-you-better-freaking-believe-it-let-me-tell-you-I'll-both-cut-to-the-chase-and-get-to-the-bottom-of-this. I'll figure it out. Perhaps, there are partners out there who are better than I am at actually getting useful, coherent information out of our medical adversaries, but other than a few random occasions, where more than anything, I was simply interpreting what my wife was having difficulty saying to a doctor, I did not fare much better. Early on, though, I was simply receiving reports from Julie of what they were telling her might or could possibly be happening.

Because of our concerns related to the irregular periods and the spotting, my wife had tests[10] done with her OB/GYN ("OB1") after October, primarily to test for PCOS. To do this, the medical facility tested her levels of insulin, testosterone, which is often elevated in people with PCOS, FSH/LH,[11] and prolactin. The results of these tests, like everything else thus far, were not terribly enlightening: Insulin and testosterone levels were "great." The insulin was "very low," which the doctor said was "perfect," so there was no need for any medication to adjust blood levels. OB1, however, did mention

---

[10] These were covered by health insurance with a moderate co-pay as they did not qualify as a fertility treatment. Thus, we're still, theoretically, in the black.

[11] "FSH/LH" is "follicle stimulating hormone/luteinizing hormone," which, from what I have been able to discern, are hormones. Whether this particular hormone is one hormone with two names, or two hormones that spend a lot of time together, or how this hormone interacts with the other many hormones splashing around in the primordial ooze that is apparently pumping rapidly through the body, I do not know. You may think me a fool or else not sufficiently conscientious that I did not actually take time or exert any effort to research and understand all of this, for lack of a better word, stuff. And you may be right. In my defense, however, I was wholeheartedly opposed to going to the Internet to "research" any medical issue. Is eHow, Yahoo! Answers, or some other POS website going to give me viable information? Is the Internet going to do anything other than cause unnecessary, hypochondriacal panic? Otherwise, in this day and age, where would I go? The library? In the end, I did still have a certain deference when it came to medicine, deference to people who presumably went to school for this and did this for a living.

that she thought the hydroxy-progesterone was "high," so she wanted an endocrinologist, a hormone doctor, take a look at it.

Sometime thereafter, we visited OB1 to learn the results of the endocrinologist's tests, and I determinedly (or else, sheepishly and pointlessly) accompanied my wife. The trip, as I remember it, was unspectacular. OB1 was busy and only stopped in for a moment. She was tall with blond hair, looked about late-thirties, or a little older. She wore running shoes and a beeper, and she actually got beeped while we were there. There were colorful doctor's scrubs. Yellow. The beep was a delivery, I believe; what else would it have been? Photos of babies lined the hallways. The woman at the front desk was a total bitch.

For the brief seconds we saw OB1, she was by no means intimidated by me. She sat quickly in the only remaining chair in our observation room, and I caught one, rapid glance into my corner. I felt that look meant she may have been just the slightest bit wary of me, wary that I might be, well, what I had hoped to be: demanding, wanting answers, wanting results, asking for something other than a quick glance over a file and then getting up to go— belligerent, perhaps. But for us, at the time, there was not much to demand. The one level of one blood test of one something that may have been high had come back and it was, "nothing to worry about" and "nothing that should inhibit fertility," although the OB did say that they might need to test it again more closely later on if we proceeded to a fertility clinic. Her recommendation at that point was more medical tests—this time, tests to determine ovulation.

So that was that: We had another step to take, which was all we could ask for, right? I thought that if we could confirm ovulation, then that would be a load off of both of our minds. That would be significant progress. We returned home.

They tested my wife's progesterone on Day Twenty-One of her next cycle (in early January 2011) to see if she had ovulated. If a woman is experiencing a typical twenty-eight-day cycle, she is supposed to ovulate on Day Fourteen-ish and the progesterone will have spiked by Day Twenty-One. (If she gets pregnant, the progesterone remains high.) This particular cycle, my wife's had not spiked—it was 0.7 (joules or megahertz, I think)—so they, the physicians or lab techs or whoever happened to be wandering by the telephone at the time, assumed that she did not ovulate. Spotting occurred again, four to seven days prior to the period's beginning, and, once the period finally arrived, it had been forty-three days since the last.

We assumed that whoever was analyzing these numbers had taken into account the significant possibility that, since Julie had irregular cycles, when she was tested, she may not have ovulated yet. Now, I'm not so sure. Perhaps instead, that particular fact was written on a medical chart somewhere, scratched in indiscernible script, sandwiched in with many others, buried in file folders, and locked in an imposing cabinet in a drab, medical office-building domino among many others off of Elliston Place in Nashville, never to see the day or help shine the light of logic on these particular numbers. But I don't know. Either way, this test didn't seem to confirm or disaffirm anything.

Based on this one month of tests though, OB1 determined that my wife was not ovulating and started her on 50 mg of Clomid, a common fertility drug, that she was to take on days five through nine of her cycle for the next three months.

This course of treatment—the Clomid for three months—was not a surprise. We were well aware that OB1 required three months of Clomid before she would refer a patient to a fertility clinic. At this point, we had no distinct desire to make it to a fertility clinic, but we also wanted to make sure that we were always moving forward. Thus, we quickly agreed to take the Clomid or anything else she recommended, because, to the extent we eventually needed to go to a fertility clinic, we wanted to be at the point where we had the referral and it was an option.

***

Throughout this process of "trying," I remember our meandering in and among different schools of thought—not necessarily highly developed and sophisticated institutions of learning, but instead, let's call them basic, unverified ideas that someone had told someone at some point after seeing something on the Internet or hearing something fourth-hand from someone else. At one point, for instance, it was presumed best that we have sex every two to three days so as to maximize sperm production. On other days—one week in particular—we were having sex every single day. Then, for a while, it was important to try to make it happen, bright and early, first thing in the morning: I believe I was woken up in the 4:30 a.m. range once before my wife had to catch a flight to New York. ("Shazzam!")[12] Then there were all of the old wives' tale tricks, such as the woman standing on her head after it was done or, essentially, while it was ongoing.

Again, with the succor of a giant, magnifying glass hindsight and a lizard with a ladder[13] I could borrow to climb up and gaze longingly back at my recent past, this wasn't such a bad way of going about doing things, because, lots of sex, bro, and little did we know, it was about to get significantly worse for a long period of time. But, because we were consumed constantly with doubt, with an aching sense that there could be something wrong such that it

---

[12] At my college fraternity, after our old cook, Hank, had been forced to retire because of ill health, we bungled around for a bit before settling on a line cook from some not particularly high-end restaurant in Charlottesville where one of my friends had been a bartender. The new cook was known eventually as Matt the Crazy Indian. Hank, on one hand, had been an icon, a major selling point to anyone, really, for the classic, Virginia fraternity experience. He had been cooking at the fraternity house for years and years and years. He was a very good cook for heavy, southern fare, but, more than anything, he was a remarkable character: a stooped but solid, older, black man with a hearty, out-of-nowhere laugh. He used to provide me a new nickname every month or so as soon as I walked in the kitchen door: "There goes old Stu…ole easy-talking Stu…ole backpack Stu…ole haircut Stu…oh, Stu." He caught me singing Pure Prairie League one time and, from then on out, it seemed, he would insist that I sing a few lines from "Amie" whenever I was walking though; when I did, he'd break into a big toothy grin. See Pure Prairie League, "Amie" (RCA, 1972). Other times, he would get serious, grip my hand in his worn, sandpapery paw, and I'd notice his eyes tearing up as he'd impart a bit of knowledge from his time on Earth. Still other times, for laughs, he would put dead squirrel carcasses against my friend Greg's bedroom window.

College provided me many moments of being too hungover to think and many other memories of being so broken by drink and alcohol-saturated anxiety that, if I could think, I was probably thinking only one thing: "I want to die." See T.S. Eliot, *The Waste Land* (The Dial Publishing Company, 1922). But these memories unfairly overshadow unique moments that cannot be found anywhere else, and one was coming over Carr's Hill after an all-day chili cook-off in which we had entered a batch of Hank's chili. It was good chili, and it won. We were fraternity pledges at the time, drunk and happy, and had been manning the chili station all day. We marched home, carrying a stereo, the prize, on our shoulders. As we crested the hill, we could see that half the fraternity and Hank were standing outside the kitchen door anxiously anticipating our arrival. There he was, a proud, unshakeable grin on his face, and we serenaded him with fraternity songs. Hank was a prankster, a storyteller, and a lover of life. Matt, on the other hand, was a nice enough guy, but cooking for a fraternity was clearly too much for him to handle. He also may or may not have had a serious drinking and drug problem. Anyway, Matt's meals devolved very quickly from set, square meals into simply lots of hot dogs. "Hot Dogs! Who wants a pot of boiling, mother-fucking hot dogs? Shazzzaaaam!" He also liked to say, "Shazzam."

[13] See *Alice in Wonderland* (Disney, 1951) ("There goes Bill." "Poor Bill.").

wouldn't matter one way or the other if I was just bombing out super sperm while she was hanging completely upside down, it made even this part of what should be an enjoyable process, at times a grind.

Of course, I'm not saying that I'm not a total effing man, y'all. But, after a month on Clomid, trying every other day, and then after another month on Clomid, trying every day, and then after another month on Clomid, saving up and trying on the most likely days imaginable, still without success, you inevitably start thinking there must be a problem here that plain old, excessive lovemaking cannot overcome. We started looking to other solutions.

Furthermore, it was through this six-months-or-so-long process that the peer-group baby boom began in force. And once my friends' wives started to get pregnant, then it made the stress—for Julie, especially—significantly worse.

I had a few equally unproductive ways of trying to deal with this concern. At one point, I was pushing the idea of stretching out our conceptual conscious timeline so that, instead of thinking on a monthly cycle where every thirty (or more) days would bring a new potent dose of disappointment and panic, we could start thinking on a year- or two-year-long cycle. That is, don't worry if you don't get pregnant this very next month; that's fine, that's OK. Just start worrying if you're not pregnant in, say, a year or, God forbid, two years. Look at the big picture! (This method met with limited success.)

Otherwise, it was extremely tough to know how to properly respond to this news that poured in month after month after month, that this new person was pregnant and that person that we had not thought about in quite a while was pregnant, and, oh, yeah, remember them, just got married, got pregnant on their honeymoon. Even, unfortunately, when it came to close friends of mine, I felt that my experience of and reaction to their happy news during what should have been a fascinating moment of the we're-so-mind-blowingly-old variety was less than admirable.

My initial response was not jealousy, because I was certainly happy for them. But, of course, I'm a man—in fact, a total effing man—so it's not like I was crowing out the window, dancing about, or rushing to buy them a gift, a bib with a clever saying, perhaps: "Party at my crib, 4:00 a.m."[14] Even more, though, than just having a stereotypically subdued masculine reaction, when hearing this news, my immediate thought was not overflowing with interest

---

[14] During the summer of 2001, my friend Luke and I did temp work in Boulder, Colorado. One job was a week-long gig sitting at a card table, facing each other, in a storage unit and, later, in the parking lot outside of the storage unit in the sun, clamping together bibs with clever sayings, onesies, and little baby booties for an eventual sale, allegedly, to J.C. Penney. "Party at my crib, 4:00 a.m." was one such saying.

and excitement for my friend, but instead went immediately to Julie and I felt just the slightest bit of resentment. Not that my friend had had the audacity to get his wife pregnant and not that he would be procreating sooner than I would be able to spread my seed out there in the world. It was because now, at this point in my particularly solipsistic existence, he had forced an unfortunate situation on *me*. I had to go tell my wife (or not, although hiding it was not usually the best course of action, either) and deal with the aftermath.

I remember when Charlie, one of my oldest, long-time, childhood friends, called to tell me his news. Once I answered, I anticipated the reason for the call pretty quickly, and I took the phone back into our bathroom and shut the door. I thought back to when Charlie had called us only a year or two before to tell us he was engaged. We were in the car on a drive up to Roanoke, Virginia, Julie's hometown. She had been shocked and immediately asked questions: "When? Where? How did it happen? This is so exciting!"

When I dropped this news on her not long after this call, she was noticeably upset, because this, among other things, seemed to be yet another potent reminder that we were losing precious time each day that went by. And of course, it was also, inevitably, a poke by the real fear that was ever-present: What if it *never* works for us? Thereafter, though, or maybe simultaneously, Julie got disappointed with herself—disappointed that she was upset, because this was joyous, happy news, and she was someone who loved babies and was happy for her friends and had never anticipated that news like this could possibly be in the slightest bit disappointing.

At this point in time, the news of our fertility struggles was certainly not public knowledge, and I had not willfully told any of my male friends. I obviously did not choose to delve into it with Charlie then, as it was not the time. Then again, I never reached out to make any time the time, either. Instead, as months went by, I felt, rather unfairly perhaps, that my friends who had pregnant wives just, fundamentally, didn't get it. I had something going on that I could not explain and did not ever attempt to explain, and they, therefore, certainly could not understand it. At the same time, they had something going on that I could not understand.

Maybe I was selling my friends short and I should have reached out to them instead of allowing a basic, subconscious resentfulness to tweak its way in. Or maybe we were just getting older and the inevitable conclusion was that friends, commiserating with friends, and confiding in friends on certain of these later-in-life adult experiences, were simply less important. Perhaps the pregnant wife marked the dividing line between before and after, between the all-important friends and then the actually important family.

Or maybe I was just clamming myself up with self-focus and sorry-feeling. Maybe you have to make an effort to put your friends into your story to help you out, because there are situations where stoicism has limits.

***

A knee-jerk reaction that doctors do not know anything and are a fabulous waste of money (although at this point, before an actual "fertility" treatment was involved, that money was theoretically just the insurance company's)[15] is not an entirely worthwhile one to have. Of course, I recognize many times over that modern medicine is great and all and something that I wholeheartedly take for granted, but it was also right around this time, February 2011, that I had occasion to take my father to the emergency room early one morning because he had a high fever and some delirium that we thought might be something worse.

One Tuesday morning, I was awakened by a call from my mother at 3:30 a.m. She was in Colorado visiting my younger sister, and Julie was out of town for work. I used my cell phone as an alarm clock, so I heard the ring and answered. My mother was upset and told me that my father had called her earlier in the night. He was not making sense, and she needed me to drive over to their house immediately. I woke up fairly quickly after that—the old floors of the bungalow creaked in the night—and made the relatively short drive down Woodmont Boulevard over Hillsboro Road to Green Hills. When I pulled in, I noticed that the outside lights and a majority of the lights downstairs were on.

Upon entering, I walked slowly, anticipating something, although I knew not what. But there was no shocking scene. I found my father, standing in the kitchen, looking relatively normal in his jammies and a robe, drinking coffee.

I said loudly, "Dad, it's Stuart. Mom called me. She said you were awake, and that I should come on over here. It's 3:30 in the morning, you know? Are you doing OK?"

He looked at me completely normally and began answering me normally, with a common start to a conversation, "Oh, well, yes," but then he quickly trailed off, "I mean, I, well…like I say…" After a moment or two, he simply looked down. The "like I say" was one of his familiar colloquialisms.

I said, "Dad, are you feeling OK? You know you probably don't need to be up and awake."

---

[15] See *Menace II Society* (New Line Cinema, 1989) ("It ain't mine.").

He looked me in the eye, but the answer again was similar, "Well, yes, of course…" Then he simply stopped talking.

I noticed that the Spanish language HBO was on the TV in the living room and *Appaloosa* with Viggo Mortensen was playing.[16] I walked in and found the remote. "Dad, you know this is—you know you're not on the right channel, right?" I then added, I'm not quite sure why, "This is *Appaloosa* with Viggo Mortensen."

"You know W.D. used to raise Appaloosa horses up in Idaho," he said. "But that, of course, was many years ago."

"Oh, really, I don't think I knew that," I said. W.D. was my dad's older brother, whom I had never met and who had died years before I was born. I changed the channel to the normal HBO. "Have you been watching this movie?" I asked.

"No, no, I don't think so," he said.

"Why don't we sit down?" He was restless, it seemed, but he took a seat at the kitchen table. "You know, I talked to Mom earlier," I said. "And she said you sounded a little confused so that's why I came over here. Are you feeling better?" There was not much of an answer.

Not long after, I walked out into the entry hall and called my mother. She told me that my dad's doctor had been paged, but he had not called back. We agreed that there was not a whole lot we could do for now, as the situation did not appear too precarious. I stuck around for a while longer and tried to get him to watch TV. After that, I left. It was still dark outside, but the birds were starting to chatter.

I drove back to Ninth Avenue, showered, and got ready for work. I was planning on maybe lying in bed, at least for an hour or so, when my mother called me again, frantic this time. She said my dad's doctor had finally called. He had expressed a fear of meningitis and that I should take him to the emergency room immediately. I got fully dressed for work quickly and raced back over to my parents' house.

Upon entering this time, I walked into the entry hall and found my dad with his head on the banister at the top of the stairs—awake but swaying and incoherent.

"Dad, are you all right?" I said. "Dad, I think we need to go to the hospital." There was no response.

I convinced him to change clothes though, and led him into his bedroom. He perked up for a second and made a joke, "You don't think I can go like

---

[16] *Appaloosa* (New Line, 2008).

this?" referring to his pajamas.

We got in the car, and I turned on sports radio. I tried to start an open-ended conversation about the Titans' off-season moves, but it was difficult. He did direct me, however, to the relevant emergency room.

After that, our experience was similar, I'm sure, to that of many others who find themselves unlucky enough to be in an emergency room at 6:00 a.m. There was a battery of tests for my father; a battery of questions regarding medications; a string of nurses or techs asking the same questions, taking the same information again and again. One of the nurses knew my dad because my dad had been practicing ophthalmology in Nashville for many years.

The ER doctor appeared at some point, wearing a West Virginia Mountaineers emblem woven into his scrubs. He was a robust man with curly gray hair and a box-shaped head. He lacklusterly ordered a test or two more before disappearing back into the hall. My older sister and brother-in-law arrived soon thereafter, carrying their infant child, and of course, inevitably, my dad started acting far more normally than he had for the previous few hours. Suddenly, our trip to the emergency room seemed an overreaction.

More time went by. As we were nearing the four-hour mark, it was apparent to all that the initial crisis had faded. It was also apparent that the ER staff was not actually expecting any answer to anything from the many tests that had apparently been taken. It was clear, in fact, that this entire transaction was essentially over.

We still found ourselves, though, all four of us plus infant, waiting in an emergency room examination room—waiting on something…not quite Godot, I guess, because in the end, it wasn't *that* long, but maybe, instead, on a West Virginia Mountaineer mascot with one of those giant, inflatable heads to appear and usher us out of the hospital in order to polish off the senselessness of the entire experience.

Eventually around 10:00 a.m., when we still, in my mind, had accomplished nothing but simply had the ER doctor call my dad's doctor with whom my mom had already been speaking, I started to feel annoyed. We had been waiting to get a final confirmation or final determination or at least permission to leave, and we weren't getting anything. In fact, no one had bothered to stop by our room in what seemed like days.

Jacked up on coffee and disrupted sleep, I walked out of the room and saw the ER doctor sitting at a computer at the central emergency room desk, laughing with a nurse next to him or in his lap or playing pussyfoot with him under the table.

I felt angry. After the fact, because my mind does not work quite this quickly, I felt that, at this point in the proceedings, I should have walked up to him, grabbed my tie, flashed it in his face in a moment of righteous verve, and said something along the lines of, "Hey, fuckface. Do you know what I'm wearing? I'm wearing a tie. That's what this is. It's a fucking tie. I don't wear a basketball jersey to work. And I'm wearing a tie, because, if you can believe it, I'm supposed to be at work *right now*, you know, 10:00 a.m. on a Tuesday!" I would then proceed to indulge my rage and tell him in grand detail with many a mellifluous curse word how important being a commercial litigator was to humanity and how each hour I spent sitting in a room waiting on nothing was one in which the world's economy was being deprived of my productivity.

Obviously, I did not make this speech. Nor did I, say, throw a cup of piss in the guy's face or anything. Instead, I asked him rather tersely if there was anything else we needed to do. He said no and that we could leave shortly. Paperwork was processed. At some point, in passing, it was finally communicated to us that there was absolutely nothing the ER could do because the issue was "viral." The best thing for my dad would be to go home and sleep and kick the fever. And, oh yeah, the doctor dropped in without much ado that it might be a bigger issue that he—along with every other doctor on the planet—couldn't actually do anything about, ever. But he wasn't sure. If it was, though, that was bad.

After some discussion, my older sister took my dad home. She called me later and said he was much better. He had insisted that she didn't need to babysit him. I went on to work.

***

So, Clomid Month One: My wife went in for a progesterone draw on Day Twenty-Four and the progesterone had spiked. It was seventeen, so apparently, she did officially ovulate on Clomid. When the period came, she had had a thirty-two-day cycle, but no pregnancy and there was still spotting. During Month Two, she had a progesterone draw on Day Twenty-Three of her cycle; it had spiked again to twenty-one and the period came on Day Twenty-Eight of the cycle. Again, ovulation. In Month Three, my wife was not able to go in until Day Twenty-Six because of another work trip. Progesterone was 5.6. She had probably ovulated and it was on its way down, but of course, there was no way of knowing because work trips had not been factored into the analysis. Rogue variable. Her period began on Day Thirty of the cycle. No pregnancy.

So, although irregularity had seemingly been overcome with the assistance of drugs, the spotting still existed. OB1 did finally acknowledge this issue and ordered an ultrasound to see if my wife had a polyp, but the ultrasound indicated no polyps or cysts on her ovaries. OB1 did see tiny follicles, though, which she said were presumably nothing to worry about, so the ultrasound still was considered "normal." She did tell us, though, that follicles are often indicative of PCOS and occur in women that are labeled "anovulatory," i.e., who cannot ovulate. Thus, apparently, PCOS was still a possibility, and although the Clomid had seemed to indicate otherwise, we still had symptoms of someone who could not ovulate.

As such, even faced with medically verifiable evidence of ovulation, we still managed to convince ourselves that, even if we were ovulating, we were not *really* ovulating, or else ovulation was not the problem. The Clomid had not solved anything. We knew that even if all these numbers seemed to say that we were OK, something, somewhere was still not quite right. And we felt, at this point, that the only way to address that something was to take a more substantial step. We believed that a fertility treatment was going to be necessary.

Thus, after Julie's three months on Clomid, OB1 gave us the referral to the Tennessee Fertility Center ("TFC").[17] In fact, a transition had occurred in our thinking and the fertility clinic had rather quickly become the goal. The TFC represented progress, not simply sitting on our hands, or else doing handstands, and hoping. We would, instead, take control of the situation and force it to happen. We thought that someone at the TFC would be able to definitively diagnose something and then fix it. We thought that, at the TFC, something would finally get done.

---

[17] Name changed.

Off Elliston Place, Nashville, Tennessee

"The Okefenokee's On Fire"

As I was not, at this point, broadcasting our troubles to any of my friends, who, in the grand scheme of conversationalists, are more amenable to enlightened discussions of porn[18] and what this says about what

---

[18] I'm hesitant to delve into pop culture commentary, for a number of reasons, but mainly because I know that so many people do it far better than I do. It'd be like taking up watercolor painting. I like to trace this realization back to my reading of one line in Anthony Lane's review of *The Phantom of the Opera* movie from 2005. Behold:

> "The irony is that, as visual habits go, there is none more threadbare than this brand of subterranean gothic, at once fussy and lumpen, with its frankly unhygienic mixture of lingerie and dungeons."

Anthony Lane, "Unmasked," *The New Yorker*, Jan. 3, 2005. That, friends, was Mike Tyson on Leon Spinks. That was Patriots–59, Titans–0 (2009) with Randy Moss catching one-handed, fifty-yard bombs in the end zone in the snow, while the Titans and their creative counterparts behind The Phantom flop around on the ground, fake an injury, and get carted away. That was a destruction in thirty-three words that, if you think about it, all major players in that movie are still attempting to overcome. One sentence of movie-reviewing perfection. (In an awkward, getting-to-know-you session in law school, the question posed to the group was: If you could do anything, any job, any profession, what would it be? I had plenty of time to think about it as I was on the far side of our Greek theatron lecture hall, but, when it came around to me, I said: "Movie reviewer." That, honestly, might have been the stupidest, sober thing I've ever said. Movie reviewer? I don't know why the obvious, inherent answer was not the first thing in my mind: professional athlete, professional soccer player in Europe, with sick tattoos up and down my arms—the first few lines of *Notes From Underground*, in Russian, emblazoned across my torso. See Fyodor Dostoevsky, *Notes From Underground* (Epoch, 1864). Or else, at the very least, movie *director*, movie *writer*. Movie reviewer?) Second, in this age of Twitter and Internet news article

it means to be human, than, say, my wife was, I wasn't able to dig deeply into what I saw as a fairly interesting sociological study: what pornography fertility centers provide for their "patients." I, happily, have only been to two fertility offices, the TFC and a doctor's office in Dallas, but there were a few notable differences between them—the primary being: TV or no TV?

In May 2011, I took my first trip to the Tennessee Fertility Center for semen-testing. I, later, in derision, referred to the TFC as a train station, and I'm not sure I was entirely wrong. It had a large office with a waiting room that probably seated forty with a decent view down Charlotte Avenue of downtown Nashville. At first, I tried to avert my eyes upon entering this spacious waiting area—ashamed to be seen, I suppose—but by the end, I ceased to care. I walked in, strutting like a fresh-steamed suit, sat in the same chair each time (Stuart's Chair!)—read my same one car magazine each time (big car fan!)—and flashed my medical bracelet after my name was called without even being asked to before being led to the beat-off wing. But the first time, of course, was different.

The nurse guided me through the first door, checked my arm bracelet, and then I followed her to the left through a set of swinging doors, only capable of being opened with a special key card. Once in, we hooked a hard right through an unlocked door into a suite of six, private rooms. I cannot say I

---

comment sections, the latter being the Fourteenth Circle of Hell—Can you imagine poor Virgil having to explain the Internet comment section Circle of Hell to Dante? "Yes, I understand the other circles are pretty bad, the traitors, the dudes gnawing each other's faces off for eternity, etc., but here, you just have to sit and listen to these fucking idiots talk forever. Believe me when I tell you, after a year or two, you'd be happy to be drowning in your own filth."—it seems clear that every asshole posting comments anywhere has got an opinion about pop culture products, and I'd rather not be one. With that said and apropos of the word "porn," I will say that I love *Love Actually* (Universal, 2003) as much as the next human being with a heart, but two parts of the movie have always been highly dissatisfying to me: (1) The entire Keira Knightley sequence, where I imagine we were supposed to think it beautiful how an obsessive, creep weirdo has been weirding out on his best friend's fiancée for months on end. (Obviously, this entire storyline has been at least partially redeemed for me once I realized that the two-bit, loser, best friend-lover, later in life, turned out to be a ruthless, blood-spattered, and now-and-then-insane, zombie killing machine in charge of a group of ragtag survivors in the zombie apocalypse—a transformation that, I must say, was unexpected); and (2) when Bill Nighy admits that he "loves" his manager—platonically, I thought—and at the climax he turns down an Elton John party to hang out with his buddy so that they can sit around, get drunk, and watch "porn." I don't know about you, and I say this having gone to an all-boys high school, but, good gracious, the days of all-male group porn watching usually ends sometime around the age of sixteen or seventeen, right? Right? And one-on-one, heterosexual, male porn-watching doesn't usually happen ever, I don't think.

ever noticed any of the other rooms being closed on any of my trips, which, in hindsight, is good for some reason, I guess. But we would proceed into one of the compartments, the nurse would give me the quick collection directions (by the end, I'd usually just give her a knowing nod), and then it would all begin.

Although writing this narrative makes me forget that anything else was going on in my life at the time, I was actually employed during all of this. On this first occasion in May, I was actually in the middle of an arbitration, where although I was at the bottom of the law firm's hierarchical totem pole, I was intimately involved in the case and the experience of even sitting through such a legal process was an incredibly valuable one. But because in any stage of the fertility process, time is of the essence—in fact, time is forever and always crumbling off the cliffside of your life in rocky chunks blown by the Nothing[19]—I *had* to fit this first semen sample in during lunch on the first day of the arbitration. So I politely darted out in order to make it back for our opening statement.

After the nurse led me into the back closet, I filled out the required worksheet: name, birth date, signature, amount of time since your last ejaculation, did you catch all of the swimmers in the plastic cup? ("Don't know yet, but I have faith that I will be able to do so."), etc. I then awkwardly crammed my name and birth date both on the lid of the cup and the cup itself, which may or may not be completely not reassuring. And here, the important differences began to shine through.

At the TFC, there is a large, brown, leather recliner and sitting on the seat of this lazy La-Z-Boy is what is, in essence, a giant, medical, paper towel, folded up nicely, in squares. There is a golf poster on the wall and classic rock plays somewhere, softly, from what I imagined was an old-fashioned AM/FM radio stashed underneath the floorboards, to provide ambient sound. And in a magazine rack by the lounge chair are two or three *Playboys* and a couple of *Penthouses*. They were periodically replaced.

In Dallas, on the other hand, there was no beat-off suite. The bathrooms were sprinkled throughout the doctor's office and were presumably used by the other patrons of the building when necessary for toileting purposes. And, although the Dallas office's magazine racks were stocked with only the *Playboys* and *Penthouses* of the world, there was also a large, flat-screen TV with a DVD player, right in the bathroom there with you. If you turned the television on, you were sent to the DVD menu of what appeared to be a fairly

---

[19] See *The NeverEnding Story* (Warner Bros., 1984) ("The neverending stooooooorrrrreeeeeeeeee. Nananananananana.").

recently produced Hustler-Vivid porno. The particular video was definitely of the same ilk as my adolescent youth—an old, nasty porno.[20]

In the end, it seems understandable that both masturbation stations do not move past *Penthouse* in the magazine realm, which means it's all naked ladies (with no dudes involved). My experience with anything beyond the staples of what counts for "respectable" magazine pornography means one would be delving into the extremely bad taste of *Hustler* or else magazines that advertise the fact that they are just "barely" abiding by the law. And, for a thousand reasons, it is readily apparent why neither group would simply provide an Internet feed.

But, in hindsight, the question arises: How did the TFC come to the decision to only have magazines? I doubt they were short on cash, so actually, why didn't they invest in a few TVs and make some nurse somewhere contact a local porn broker and pick up some of the latest vids? And when and how was a decision made? Was there a board meeting? Who keeps the meeting minutes? Was this the CEO's call? Did one of the doctors object vociferously and argue that videos are simply unnecessary and any pornography whatsoever with a man involved is demeaning to women? Was there a discussion? And why was Dallas more casual about it? Were they—in Texas—just more mature about the whole thing, less Puritan than the Tennesseans? Did Dallas make a conscious decision not to segregate the masturbators? Did Dallas have a better understanding of the human condition?

Or, more likely, no one out there in the world thinks too much about it, or maybe, at the TFC, they assume that if you cannot get it going the old-fashioned, magazine way, then you've got your own problems. Or maybe the TFC did make a conscious decision that it would have no full penetration, just to be polite. I simply don't know. But, if you spend enough time rolling around beat-off closets with your pants down, such strains of thought eventually take a turn spinning pointlessly through your mind.

In the end, my only brief bit of advice is that—this is the self-help portion of this narrative, so please pay attention—if you're wearing a suit, just go ahead and take the pants off entirely and hang them up. You should keep your socks on, needless to say, but waddling around with your pants around your ankles, holding a plastic cup, desperately hoping to catch all that is necessary into the container so that you won't have to admit failure on the form you must fill out after it is all said and done, is tough. But, yes, punch it out. Seal that lid. Press the magic "I voted" button (alerting the nurses behind the wall that the

---

[20] See, e.g., *Fever* (no citation information available).

specimen is primed and ready), and then be gone out the side door. Let them bill you for it later. [$125 for the initial semen-testing.][21]

The TFC was like a train station, though, or maybe a bus station, complete with freaks in back rooms with their pants off and marked by a seemingly constant influx and exodus of downtrodden folks, clutching their spouses and moving rapidly in different directions. Women are quietly shuffled into side rooms, while the men are stranded outside in a hallway, despondent and alone, but always, people moved in one door, moved out another, key cards swiped, blood drawn, names called, frowns. In such numbers, in fact, that I had to marvel at the sheer volume of individuals (all with fertility problems?) and the copious amount of revenue those people represented for a place that did not have to deal with insurance companies or reduced reimbursement rates or co-pays, but were simply paid in full right then and there after each exam, each IUI, each IVF, each prescription, each visit, each specimen collection. Pure commerce being pumped in and out. So, train station? Maybe not—more like a casino where the house never has to pay out.

So alas, after the third failed round of Clomid and the vaginal ultrasound that indicated a possible presence of a uterine polyp—a hazy ultrasound image of something that could have been nothing, diagnosed by OB1 who couldn't really tell—we were referred to the TFC. The TFC, at that time, had four physicians, and the one doctor recommended to us by a friend had a month-long wait, which once we saw the TFC's constantly rotating turnstile, was not terribly surprising. We opted for another, Dr. X (hereinafter, "Fertility Doctor" or "FD"). We had our first appointment with her at the TFC on May 13, 2011 [$20 co-pay for initial visit, because the TFC coded the meeting as one related to the alleged polyp and not strictly for fertility purposes.]

This time, unlike my previous visit with OB1, there was a significant amount of pent-up emotion and frustration present and boiling under a bouncing lid. It had been nine months of constant trying, which meant it had been nine months of constant insecurity and uncertainty. Nine months of wandering around pointlessly, juggling a soccer ball with no lines, no goal, no players, just periodically turning and kicking as far as we could, just to race after it a bit later and discover that we were still standing in an empty field. So, on this trip, we were looking for progress, and progress for us was a diagnosis and a clear course of action. Something different.

The Fertility Doctor arrived with my wife's file—a relatively hefty one for not having been definitely diagnosed with any treatable problem. She was

---

[21] The tab officially starts running now.

probably in her late forties or early fifties, with dark hair pulled back tight, attractive but maybe cold—the gleaming, white, alternate-timeline-Ghost-of-Christmas-Future, Karen Allen in *Scrooged* springs to mind.[22] The FD had clearly not reviewed the file until that moment. I noticed that, but shrugged it off at the time. I was maintaining hope that the FD would actually have answers, and thus, I was assuming, perhaps, that doctors always wait to review new patient files until the moment they are actually, physically crossing the threshold into the room where the patient happens to be waiting. That's just how it works. The consultation room was windowless with a 3-D rendering of a uterus. We began telling our story, or Julie did: the details of the irregularity, the spotting, the Clomid, the verified ovulation, and she immediately became upset.

I attempted to jump in. I knew most of the details and filled them in where I could. "Maybe a polyp," I said. "We still have some concerns about PCOS," I added later. "We think ovulation definitely did happen, but then again, we're not sure."

After listening to our initial tale and after a brief glance at my wife's file, the FD did at this point look and stare at what seemed like a point directly past Julie's head and said, point-blank, "You will get pregnant." Period. That statement in and of itself was comforting. It was something I would bring up to my wife and periodically repeat in the months to come—hollow support, perhaps, once you begin to realize that it may have been the equivalent of someone speeding by while your car is broken down on the side of the road (or in a ditch, on fire) and shouting, "Oh, it'll start!"—but some comfort, nonetheless.

The FD then laid out the course of action. (She had a notepad facing us, and she was writing upside-down. When she was done jotting down pertinent details, she continued blindly doodling curlicues). She recommended we move to IUIs (intra-uterine inseminations) while switching to the drug Femara to induce ovulation. Clomid apparently can dry up one's "cervical fluid," making it difficult for sperm to travel.[23] The FD wanted us to try Femara, a breast cancer drug that they found caused women to ovulate, so its use as fertility medicine was off-label. She said women typically produce fewer eggs

---

[22] See *Scrooged* (Paramount, 1988).

[23] Thereafter and for the foreseeable future, insufficient cervical fluid became another closet monster we were previously unaware of that had my wife testing her "fluid" and trying to diagnose its presence, potency, or lack thereof, for some time to come. She simultaneously began consuming strangely large volumes of non-drowsy cough syrup, which an old wives' tale told us increased cervical fluid.

on Femara, so the risk of conceiving multiples is lower. She also added that women with PCOS are very responsive to Clomid and ovulation-inducing medications, so the risk of multiples is usually very high.

How any of this made me feel, I'm not sure. Seeing as how I didn't know what Clomid did to the body and/or the cervical fluid and/or the fact that it caused a higher risk of "multiples," I suppose I wasn't about to raise objections to an off-label use of a different drug that I, likewise, knew nothing about but apparently reduced the risk of "multiples." Sounded good.

In regard to the spotting, the FD did finally have some sort of explanation for what it could be: a "luteal phase defect," i.e. "you are a werewolf (werewolf-type)," which apparently meant that my wife was not producing adequate progesterone post-ovulation, so the uterine lining was beginning to shed too early. This meant that a theoretical fertilized egg could have been formed, but was sloughed off before it had time to implant because of a hormone imbalance. But again, she wasn't sure.

She performed an ultrasound on my wife to see if the uterine polyp the OB may have seen was visible. She and Julie made a quick trip from consultation room to examination room. I stayed in a second, interior lobby outside the examination room with a few other hapless fellows for a few minutes.

The FD did not find any polyps, but still thought that my wife probably did have PCOS due to the tiny cyst formations that she also saw on the ovaries. She did discover, however, that my wife's uterine lining looked "great" right now and that, well, she was about to ovulate!

On the ultrasound, she saw a 16mm sized follicle (an egg, about to drop), which was Day Eighteen of her cycle. Apparently, the follicles are usually considered mature when they are in the low-twenties, so this was almost there. Her thought was that there was probably still Clomid in her system (it apparently has a long half-life, again, something about which I was entirely unaware) and that was why Julie was ovulating on her own. She told us to buy a specific, over-the-counter ovulation predictor kit, [ClearBlue Easy: $25], and to call her office once Julie received a positive test.

We left the office excitedly and did as we were told. On Sunday, May 16, Julie had a positive result, so the IUI was scheduled for that following Monday, May 17. My wife was supposed to go to New York for a work trip that Monday and canceled it at the last minute.

***

If IUIs had a family crest, it would be a picture of a pipette. (The family motto: "I'm gonna get all up in there.") As I understood it at that time, the man beats off in a closet. The techs at the TFC "clean" the sperm and pick out the most promising of the million little swimmers—you know what I mean, right? Neither did I, but apparently they're looking for the ones that are shaped the best, move around the most, and have a big impressive and showy tail. It's the NFL combine for millions of sperm, just without the skin-tight pants (the mere mention of which is, of course, a fundamental faux pas in any discussion of fertility, sperm, or sperm count).

Once the best of the best are chosen, the wife arrives, gets into stirrups, and the spermies are pipette-ed into the uterus, so that the distance to travel is much shorter and more manageable and maybe the lack of viscous cervical fluid does not lead to gridlock, breakdown, and general sperm confusion. It's like Eddie Valiant popping off a few rounds on his old, cartoon gun but wasting the tomahawking Indian on a liquor bottle while the rest of the old gunslinger bullets get confused and take a wrong turn going after the villain.[24] That's what we were trying to avoid: Pick the best (just the Indian) and jam it in there forcefully so as to avoid any mix-up. Theoretically, IUIs are a solution to a problem you didn't know existed: the hurdle between ejaculation and conception.

***

I took my second trip in as many weeks to the TFC, about an hour before my wife, to provide a sample. Then, they put the cleaned and glossed, five-star spermies into a syringe attached to a thin piece of plastic tubing that they "snaked up" inside her—their phrasing—depositing the sperm into the uterus. The sperm numbers were good for quantity, motility, morphology, medicine ball reps, and whatever else they look for. According to Julie, the procedure is relatively painless—if, obviously, horribly uncomfortable and tiresome as they have the woman lie down for fifteen minutes following the insemination (so as to better harness the awesome power of gravity). We made sure to have sex the next day per their instructions with a fifteen-minute, post-coital layabout, and then we flew to Jacksonville for Julie's cousin's wedding. [IUI: $206 (male portion) + $240 (female) = $446.]

After the weekend trip, my wife had a progesterone test performed on May 23. It was 11.9 (Richter Scale, I think). Low for purposes of conception, but still in the range they wanted to see. On May 27, she started spotting. She

---

[24] See *Who Framed Roger Rabbit?* (Touchstone Pictures, 1988).

called the TFC, and they put her on 200mg of Prometrium [$25], which is a progesterone supplement in the event her progesterone was dropping off too early and causing the uterine lining to shed and lose the fertilized egg. She was to take it for four days. She had a couple of days' reprieve from the spotting on May 29 and 30, but it picked up again on May 31. Her period began June 3, 2011. The first IUI was officially unsuccessful.

At that time, the FD wanted Julie to have a hysteroscopy[25] and laparoscopy[26] to see what was causing the spotting and to check for endometriosis, another possible problem.[27] We, at that point, were certainly not not going to agree. We scheduled the procedure for Thursday, June 16.

Obviously, the failure of the first IUI was disappointing, but perhaps we knew that this problem was not going to be solved this "quickly" and "easily," and the fact that the FD was gung-ho about trying something else, something new, and something bold and/or drastic was encouraging, because answers again, appeared to be on the horizon. This seemed like a procedure by which we could actually eliminate one of these many maladies that had been loitering about. We would see if in fact endometriosis was the issue and was the cause of our troubles, and we would likewise get a final answer on the spotting. Although, to be honest, at this point, I could no longer keep track of what my wife supposedly had or did not have: probably PCOS, but maybe not. Ovarian cysts? Progesterone deficiency? But she was ovulating. Endometriosis?

***

In telling a story of attempted creation of life, I feel inclined to tell stories of loss. Fortunately, I have not experienced a terribly large number of monumental tragedies in my young life, and, if we're talking about the shocking death of a young person, I have experienced only one.

David, a college friend, the first true college friend I met my first moment in my first year suite at UVa, died tragically in 2006 while in his first year of medical school at Harvard. He had taken two girls from a bar to the rooftop of his apartment building to look at the view and had offered to put their purses

---

[25] Dilate cervix, insert flashlight/camera up through the vagina, look around. See Julie Vargo & Maureen Regan, *A Few Good Eggs: Two Chicks Dish on Overcoming the Insanity of Infertility,* 141-42 (Regan Books, 2005).

[26] Insert flashlight/camera through belly-button, then make incision below navel, insert tools and zap endometriosis. See Ibid., 142.

[27] Endometrial tissue that typically lines the uterus starts growing on other organs where it is not supposed to be. Egg gets confused, leaves uterus. See Ibid., 24-25.

in his room. He was not drunk, as he had just finished working a shift and had only been out for a little while. As he climbed down what was apparently a precarious fire escape, he slipped and fell several stories to his death.

I worked at a major law firm in New York City at the time as a woefully overpaid, terribly underutilized paralegal. I did next to nothing, every day, all day. To that point in my life, I had made a career out of that particular skill. In my first four years out of college, at my two longest tenured jobs, my primary purpose seemed to be reading the newspaper every day and playing on the Internet and getting paid (relatively) decently for it.

While at this particular job, I was already set on going to law school and, therefore, was not suffering from the constant itch/debilitating alcoholic depression/desire to do something different and great that I felt in my first two years out of college while living in Washington, D.C. Thus, I was OK with the fact that I read Bill Simmons for a living. But I worked in a small, windowless, hallway office with a great roommate, Trevor, and he and I would hang out most of the day, talking sports.

Which is what I was doing when I received a call from a college friend, Greg, who did not usually call me. I thought nothing of it. I answered. He told me there had been an accident and that David was dead. I remember that moment vividly, although I don't really remember any of the details: the computer screen, white board, or desk. I just remember that moment in time, and how I had assumed a car accident. A flash of David's car appeared in my mind, of helping him move out of his New York City apartment not long before. You don't necessarily know, or at least I hadn't thought at that time, about how I would react to tragic news; mind-blowing, shocking, completely unexpected, tragic news. For me it was nothing notable. It was overwhelming and immediate and I cried. Trevor politely left the room.

I rode to Ohio a few days later for the funeral with my friend Luke, whose boss had loaned him a car for the occasion. I made a CD for the trip: Pearl Jam's "Oceans,"[28] followed by Mason Jennings's *Use Your Voice*[29] album. I knew Luke would love the Mason Jennings and, as for the "Oceans," during our first year in college, David and I lived in a suite together and would have many, long, Nintendo 64 sessions. Each time, we'd cobble together a Winamp playlist. A few songs always made the cut: "Oceans," "Nookie,"[30] "Hit 'Em

---

[28] Pearl Jam, "Oceans" (Epic, 1992).

[29] Mason Jennings, *Use Your Voice* (Architect Records, 2004).

[30] Limp Bizkit, "Nookie" (Flip/Interscope, 1999).

Up,"[31] "Soul to Squeeze."[32] A distinct memory of comfort associates with that
SMK,[33] FIFA,[34] Oceans, and Nookie. "Oceans," in particular, on this occasion,
seemed to speak for itself.

Through the funeral process and afterward, my apparent search for
meaning from all of this gave rise to a variety of different thoughts, what I
thought were certain semi-profound insights. I thought the most interesting
was the amount of ego involved in funerals—egos of everyone else still living,
who want to claim something unique and individual that no one else could
understand, a connection with the deceased that is not sullied by repetition.
Instead, it was something that marked you, the one living, as special, as
someone who would have been treasured highly had the dead been floating
over, remembering friends.

I experienced this ego even with the loss of my maternal grandmother at
the age of ninety-one. She was the matriarch, a woman who had had a full life,
with a full family, fully loved by all. But even then different people clung to her
in different ways, and there was a surprising amount of ownership involved.
Here, it was particularly more acute because my friend David was so young,
the death was so shocking, and he himself had been especially good at moving
between diverse groups. So, after the funeral, at a big dinner in the downstairs
dining room of a surprisingly sophisticated Canton, Ohio, restaurant, I, drunk,
came treacherously close to Zinedine Zidane-ing[35] the Queen of the IMPs[36]
in an act of egomaniacal glee because I thought she was an idiot who knew
nothing and certainly knew nothing about David.

Then, several months later, I found myself at a Counting Crows concert, of
all places, in Atlanta. During one of their more emotional songs,[37] I had tears
streaming down my face. My friend Taylor's girlfriend noticed and I think
she thought I was pulling off a fairly elaborate joke about being emotionally
overcome by a Counting Crows song. But I found myself plunging into the
whole experience, and I couldn't help but think two things: (1) When he
slipped, I hoped he hadn't been scared. Knowing him, he more than likely
wasn't. I bet he thought he'd be fine. That, to me, was a good thing. (2) I hoped

[31] 2pac feat. Outlawz, "Hit 'Em Up" (Death Row, 1996).
[32] Red Hot Chili Peppers, "Soul to Squeeze" (Warner Bros., 1993).
[33] Super Mario Kart (Nintendo 64, 1997).
[34] FIFA 99 (Nintendo 64, 1998).
[35] See 2006 World Cup Final.
[36] A lower rung, UVa secret society made up, in my day, of non-major sport athletes and people in the University tour guide service.
[37] Counting Crows, "Holiday in Spain" (Geffen, 2002).

that he was then—several months after his death—a nice clean and sleek skeleton, not anything else.

I do struggle now with the concept, the real tragedy, of irrelevance, with thoughts of his inevitably being irrelevant. It's something you can't help but think and something that seems legitimate: that David knows nothing about iPhones, he knows nothing about Barack Obama, he knows nothing about his friends having children, his friends even getting married. I try to move past that, though, because even if it is a true and complete fact, it's also one that can be understood and overcome. Thus, even if you do not want to lean toward comforting thoughts that he *does* know about all of those things, even if he doesn't, to be frank, who gives a shit? It is something that you can quickly and easily forgive him for.

And, although this is definitely another completely self-conscious attempt to bring meaning here, I do try to look back on this one particular experience as an important event in my life. A horrible tragedy that made me, I think, better—not that I wouldn't trade it, of course, to recover my friend, I suppose it's worth saying, although I don't know why it's worth saying—in fact, it's not worth saying—because there simply is no trading to be done. But I do feel that this event made me wiser. I feel as if wisdom, whatever bits have attached themselves to me over time, have only been collected in little specks, over many, long months of routine and daily waking life.[38] David's death, I like to think, spurred this process along for me and, thus, was meaningful, productive in some small way.

But, of course, in the end, loss still remains. David had seemed wiser, far wiser than I certainly was, but wiser than most at our age. He was someone who had, on several different occasions in college, when things didn't matter, seemed to do small things that did. He convinced several friends of ours to take rebel flags off their walls. He never told them to do it. He never shamed them into it. He just sat them down and explained that the flag made certain people uncomfortable and that he knew that our friends might not have meant to offend anyone or make anyone uncomfortable, but under the circumstances, it might be best to err on the side of caution. Or the one time I ever got a red card in an intramural, indoor soccer game, where I found myself engaged in a fistfight with the opposing team's goalie: As the fight was broken up, after the goalie had successfully pinned my head on the basketball gymnasium floor,

---

[38] —or, better yet, the process is the opposite, one in which time removes dark, distracting globs that have always been with me and, like the *Princess Mononoke* (Miramax, 1997) ancient beast god rolling along through fields and forests, dark specks of matter are gradually sloughed off to unveil the true creature underneath—

I could see that David had jumped right in the middle and was holding both sides at bay. He was a natural peacekeeper. You had to wonder about someone like that who seemed already preternaturally wise for his age. What could he have accomplished with his life?

***

Prior to the surgery my wife had to have an HSG (hysterosonogram) performed to make sure her tubes were clear. She went to a special diagnostic facility where they inserted a catheter into her uterus so that they could inject dye and take pictures. [$166 with insurance.] The dye traveled to the fallopian tubes so the doctor could see if they were clear and determine whether or not she had any polyps or fibroids[39] that may have been blocking them and preventing conception. You might remember from sex education class or *Look Who's Talking* that the egg travels from the ovaries through the fallopian tube to the uterus and anxiously awaits one little spermie to break through the ranks and stick it in there.[40] A blocked fallopian tube could have been yet another cause of infertility. The HSG, however, came back clear and everything looked great. Julie went to two baby showers that weekend.

The surgery occurred on June 16, 2011. [$350.43 to TFC; $663.75 to the surgery center.] We were told to be there at 8:30 a.m. for the 10:30 a.m. surgery. As most people do, I try to avoid hospitals and surgical centers. When I do find myself in such a place, however, I find it odd that the clientele is almost always the exact opposite of what I would call urban sophisticates.

I remember in one particular waiting room, an older, probably seventy-year-old woman, one of about thirty people in the room, was playing some sort of game on her iPhone, the general purpose of which appeared to be killing zombies, apparently with a rocket launcher. Whatever it was, though, she seemed to be accomplishing the purpose well. She had the volume of her phone maxed out to the point that it sounded as if she were plugged into the waiting-room speaker system and a constant, incessant sound of exploding flesh reverberated. Here, there was nothing quite so flabbergasting, but needless to say, I did not feel as if I were in the environment for sipping artisan cocktails.

We arrived at 8:30 a.m., ready to go, ready to have whatever needed to be done done. We filled out pointless forms—you don't already have all of our

---

[39] I have no idea what a fibroid is.

[40] See *Look Who's Talking* (Tri-Star, 1989).

information?—which did not take terribly long, and my wife got wrapped in a dressing gown and propped on pillows on a hospital bed. In the end, though, two hours seemed a bit overzealous for our surgery "preparation."

In this particular surgery center, we did not have an individual room, just curtained-off prepping stations where we and many others waited for our respective doctors to show. With my wife dolled up in a hair net, I passed the time by admiring the air heating system that allowed warm air to be pumped into Julie's dressing gown so she got puffed up like a delicious marshmallow man. Then, well, we sat. After that, we sat longer.

My wife was good-natured. They had not given her anything at that point, but I thought she was already acting spaced out, while trying to keep a positive attitude. Or maybe I just always thought she looked fun and that her facial features were highlighted as delicate and refined when she was wearing headwear. Here it was a hospital hairnet, of course, rather than a Swedish Helga ski hat, which I would have preferred.

She was ready to go, though, and the anesthesiologist had already come by and introduced himself. Various nurses would periodically peek in on us or fluff our pillows, and our curtain would occasionally blow open, so that I could see other nurses sitting and chatting in front of a computer or an old man being wheeled by to his doom. But 10:30 a.m. was long past and we were moving closer to noon.

At this point I did perhaps intuit something—context clues or existential aura—from the two nurses outside of our station that the delay was occurring because our doctor had not shown up yet. By glimpses, various words, and glances, it became clear that this was not the first time that this particular FD had left a patient hanging. Looks of sympathy from the staff became more common.

Of course, I could have been royally annoyed, but there was no viable outlet. Unlike my experience with my father, here we were actually waiting on something significant, a medical procedure to take place. I could have, perhaps, bitched at a nurse for no reason or fashioned a hysterical speech in my mind for the woman that was about to cut my wife open. In the end, though, it seemed to make more sense to just casually sit there, responding to work messages that were not all that pressing, and continue hoping that this would be the answer to our fundamental problem.

Inevitably, our doctor did arrive—it was past 1:00 p.m., maybe even 1:30 p.m. She had a hurried excuse which I didn't believe and don't remember.[41]

---

[41] Oops the monkey had escaped from the Mill Mountain Zoo, I think.

The anesthesiologist came back and started talking to my wife while hooking up liquid bags. The hospital bed began moving, I awkwardly hugged her, and then she was gone.

My options in the waiting room were sitting and listening to fellow concerned family members watch daytime TV and slurp Sonic or nothing, so I left and went to Samurai on Elliston Place, ate sushi at the bar, and read the *Nashville Scene*.

I returned to the waiting room around 2:30 p.m. and sat for another hour. After most all others in the room were gone, I was finally called into a consultation room with one door leading in and a second door leading out in the opposite direction. I imagined that this had been arranged this way so that the doctor could enter from the dark goblin passageway beyond, while the loved one, me, was pushed in, disarmed and clueless, ready to be shot,[42] but maybe I was letting my mind wander.

Prior to the surgery, I had been schooled by Julie to ask many questions of the doctor when I finally got her in a room alone. I had not written any of the appropriate questions down, but I felt that I instinctively would know them and would perform under pressure: Was there enough evidence of endometriosis to cause fertility problems? Was this the problem? Where was the endometriosis? Did you get it all? How soon can we start trying again? Will it come back? How soon? Did it work?

Of course, when the moment arrives, the questions aren't that simple and the answers aren't that apparent. The FD had photographs of the endometriosis itself on different parts of my wife: interior human organs with slight evidence of spots, but none on the reproductive system. She zapped them. But the endometriosis was not terribly bad, although it was certainly there, yes. I tried to ask her if it was the primary issue, and I think she tried to say that it was, or at least, while not terrible, the endometriosis was there and we got it, which was the point, right? And then she was gone.

I believe later she said that it was the "perfect amount" of endometriosis, which I think meant just enough to cause some problems but not an insane amount to be *too* problematic. She classified it as "Stage Two Endo." Of course, later, the Dallas doctor said there is no such thing as a perfect amount of endometriosis, but then again, the FD had said there was certainly no polyp and that OB1 clearly had been wrong, so this was just another stop on a cross-county version of Telephone: Healthcare Edition. I also learned later that women with endometriosis have babies all the time, and, if it's a Caesarean,

---

[42] See Harold Pinter, *The Dumb Waiter* (Samuel French Ltd, 1960).

they just zap it all away after the birth while they're in there. But again, progress was better than no progress. We got the endometriosis!

I was finally allowed back to see my wife. She was the last of the surgical patients. The lights were dim in the back, the curtains from the individual waiting beds had been pulled aside and exposed, and only one nurse remained. Julie was clearly struggling out of her anesthesia and, for some reason, not terribly happy with me. Perhaps I thought that after my long day in the waiting room (or make that, eating at the best sushi restaurant in town), worrying about my poor, incapacitated wife, we would have a passionate reunion. But she was, instead, supremely annoyed.

"Did you ask her what we talked about?" she asked.

"Yes, definitely," I responded, "Of course. I mean, she gave me photos and she said we definitely, you know, got it."

In actuality, the conversation with the FD was more like:

"You know, we definitely want to start trying again immediately, if possible." That's me.

The FD said, "Of course."

I said, "So, I mean, we obviously hope this worked. This is what you think is the problem, right?"

And she said, "It was certainly endometriosis. Almost a perfect amount." She showed me pictures.

"OK, but we got it. It worked?"

"Oh yes, we definitely got it," she said.

Julie, even in her haze, seemed to know what had actually happened and that I was, well, FOS. But she had had enough of being there, and I, of course, didn't blame her. So even though she was drinking orange juice out of a straw, she was ready to go. The one nurse left on staff wanted to make sure Julie urinated before we left, but it was clear the nurse could be convinced otherwise, as she apparently wanted to leave as much as we did. We wheeled my wife over to the bathroom, and I joined her inside as she removed some bloody bandages and attempted to pass something out. Maybe the tiniest of tinkles, but, yeah, something, sure. The nurse agreed to let us go. She did also, thankfully, agree to wheel Julie downstairs as I pulled the car around. It was dusk; the work day was over. We loaded her into my car. I suppose for a flash of a moment I thought about eventually driving her home from the hospital with a tiny baby in tow or maybe, driving her to the hospital about to burst and how I would need to drive especially conscientiously, like today. We rode home uneventfully.

[We were later additionally billed $147.55 for anesthesia plus $453.75 for the surgery. Insurance covered the rest.]

***

We had moved at this point out of 12 South to Green Hills. West End Avenue moves out of downtown, past Vanderbilt, past I-440 (the interstate loop around the city) and continues west, as a variety of different neighborhoods branch off of its lifeline to both the right and left: Sylvan Park, Green Hills, Hillwood, Belle Meade, West Meade, eventually, over a hill and farther away, Bellevue.

We moved to a slightly larger home with a little backyard and a creek in the back on a cut-through street between Estes Road and Abbott Martin Road, right on the edge of Belle Meade. I had spent part of my adolescence in this general area. My high school was around the corner. I am certain I used our current street to avoid back-ups, and I am sure I sped religiously. Now if we are ever out walking at any time of day when high schoolers catapult by in their SUVs and trucks, rushing headlong and careless through our little neighborhood, we shake an angry fist and growl. One of our neighbors has put up a red and white sign that says, "Drive like your kids live here."

***

A few days after the surgery, Julie gathered more useful information—more than likely from a phone call to the TFC [$25 / call on the weekend.] The FD said the next six months were "pivotal" for us to get pregnant as the "endo" could grow back…at any moment! So, really try this time. No screwing around. When you're sending them out there, Stuart, try to keep them focused. Remember that; remember it good when you go into the beat-off closet next time. No spillage!

She recommended we stick with the IUIs, but for the next three, we were not going to use the OTC OPKs (over-the-counter, ovulation predictor kits, OC [of course.]) but rather an Ovidrel trigger shot that would force the eggs that developed from the Femara to drop. You see, Femara helps the eggs develop, and the trigger shot forces the eggs to drop directly before the IUI inserts the swimmers.

Unfortunately though, after the surgery, it took a long while for Julie's period to return. We went to St. Simons, Georgia, for the Fourth of July. My brother-in-law Tack and I got drunk and made up a song called, "The Okefenokee's On Fire," because the Okefenokee Swamp (in South Georgia) was, apparently, on fire. We went to trivia night at a local bar with the whole family and named our team "The Okefenokee's on Fire…and So Is My Crotch" (his idea). Grommets were selling new-born, eyes-still-glazed-in-blindness puppies at the end of the boardwalk at East Beach. (Come to the blazing-hot beach; buy a newborn puppy! Fresh from the womb!) Casey Anthony got acquitted.

When this news was brought up, we were jammed in a car with Julie's sister Catherine and Tack with my father-in-law driving. The verdict came in over the radio.

I said, "I, honestly, don't care."

"You don't care?" Julie asked.

"No, not really," I responded.

"Well, that's great."

"No, I mean, I obviously think it's horrible, and I, of course, care about dead kids. But, you know, people, kids, die every day, across the globe in bad ways. This was a terrible situation involving horrible rednecks, but it's gotten far more press than it deserves." I had been drinking.

Julie said, "Well, I think that makes you sound like a jerk."

The next day, I caught a tiny blue fish.

Finally, the FD prescribed my wife Prometrium again (progesterone) to kick-start her period. She was to take it for ten days and then wait for the period to come. She took it July 5 through 14 and then her period arrived July 20, 2011. The last period had been June 3, so, fifty days later, we started again.

***

Round One with Femara: We were instructed to take Femara Days Three to Seven of my wife's cycle. On August 3, 2011, my wife went to the TFC for an ultrasound and had two mature follicles. They gave her the Ovidrel shot, and we had the IUI the following day, August 4, our fourth wedding anniversary. I would give you more rich detail about my third trip to the beat-off closet, but I feel I might lose my audience. [$104.99 (Ovidrel shot); $220 (ultrasound); $206 (swimmer cleaning); $240 (insemination) = $770.99.]

On August 15, my wife got her period.

At this point, Julie started acupuncture twice a month—at times it shifted to three or four times a month. [$70 per visit for the foreseeable future.][43] I started reading *War and Peace*[44] and training for the New York City marathon.[45] I had always wanted somewhere in the back of my mind to do both of these things. In hindsight, the fact that I launched into them, simultaneously, at this particular time, is not terribly surprising, as they were seemingly important tasks that I could actually accomplish.

Newt came up with the idea for the marathon somewhat out of the blue. He had a connection through his work to a charity for homeless children, and, if we guaranteed $3,000 apiece raised for the charity, we could avoid the New York City marathon lottery and secure a spot in the race. Now seemed as good a time as any.

Round Two with Femara: Took Femara Days Three through Seven. Ultrasound on August 26. Ovidrel shot. IUI was that Saturday Aug. 27 [$770.99], right before my wife went to another baby shower.

We discussed these baby showers on multiple occasions:

"You know, you really don't have to go to these, or, at least, you don't have to stay the whole time," I said. I thought that if it were a close enough friend, she would know what was going on and would certainly understand. And if the friend wasn't as close, a quick appearance would be acceptable.

"Yes, I do," she responded.

"I mean, at the very least, you don't have to host them every time," I said.

"That's just not the way it works," Julie said.

"Well, I just imagine it's probably pretty difficult."

"It's fine."

I think, in the end, in my mind at least, baby showers were just so intense, so over-the-top for people like us, who were ensconced deep in the fertility process, that maybe she just zoned out and was numb to the whole thing. In retrospect, I doubt that is actually what happened.

Her period came September 10.

Around that time, we discovered that my sixty-year-old, maternal uncle Bill, a vibrant, life-loving, crazy-in-the-best-of-ways man, a father of five daughters who had started his own business which had grown to several hundred employees and into a major operation, had been diagnosed with metastatic melanoma—skin cancer—that had spread throughout his body, including his brain.

Round Three with Femara: Took Femara Days Three through Seven. On

---

[43] We'll call it $2,000 even.

[44] Leo Tolstoy, *War and Peace* (The Russian Messenger, 1869).

[45] I finished one of these long before the other. Guess which.

September 21, my wife had an ultrasound. Everything was ready to go once again—Follicles ready! Looks perfect! Everything is in place!—so she took the Ovidrel shot. We had the IUI the next day on Sept. 22 [$770.99], and then flew to Detroit that evening to visit my uncle.

We had a huge family gathering, touring my uncle's business operation, riding motorcycles, eating authentic Mexican food, and drinking Michigan beers. We watched converted-to-DVD 8 mm films that my grandfather had taken in Guam after the War. After the parents went to bed, all of us adult cousins stayed up late in my uncle's garage, lounging on exercise bikes and the hoods of cars. I rapped the first few verses of "Black Steel in the Hour of Chaos" by Public Enemy.[46] We partied.

But, that night, back in our room at the Hampton Inn with a glow from the parking lot light slicing through a break in the curtains, while getting ready for bed, Julie said, "This is all just so sad."

Huh? I thought. I obviously knew it was sad, but I thought that was something we would consider later. We were plucking the day. Tonight was fun. He had looked fine.

"You just think about all those girls and who's going to walk them down the aisle," she said.

I knew Julie had always loved that moment at our wedding. I just hadn't really been thinking about any of that. I was thinking about having to wake up for our flight.

"Yeah," I said. "You're right, of course."

Round Four with Femara: Took Femara Days Three through Seven. Had ultrasound October 17, had a 2 mm follicle. Ovidrel shot. IUI on the 18th. [$770.99.] You know the old Einstein quote, "Insanity is paying to beat off in a closet five times?" Well, that was, literally, exactly what this was like.) My wife started spotting on October 28 and started her period on October 31. I ran the New York City Marathon on November 4.

***

Julie and I stayed with my friend Greg and his wife on the Upper East Side. I did not sleep terribly well, probably because I was so concerned about sleeping, getting sleep, not getting enough sleep, and/or being sure to wake up at 4:00 a.m. I also knew my Uncle Bill was in hospice at that time. My mother had made the drive from Nashville to Detroit and back several times in the

---

[46] Public Enemy, "Black Steel in the Hour of Chaos" (Def Jam, 1989).

past few weeks. I didn't really know much of the details, but I did expect a call at any time.

I had a vague notion of talking to Newt during the race about both our fertility struggles and everything that had been going on with my uncle. I figured it would be an opportune time to do so, running side-by-side for many hours. Newt was married, but children seemed far off his radar, so I thought that would make him a good candidate to discuss all of this fertility business, as he would seemingly have no vested interest. He also had a tendency to have an atypical stance on many conventional matters.

Newt told me the day before, though, that he was going to try to qualify for the Boston Marathon, which, for our age, meant running a marathon in a little over three hours. I was doubtful that Newt was physically capable of doing this.

"Three hours? I mean, is that a joke?" I said. We were wandering the Jacob Javits Convention Center, packed with excited people. "Have you been training at that pace?"

"No, not really," he responded. I was also a little doubtful that Newt had been following any legitimate training regimen at all. He had previously run a marathon, years ago in college, so I think he thought he was fine.

"So what makes you think—"

"Did you bring any warm clothes?" he asked. Multiple people, including my father, who ran the New York City Marathon in 1987 in 3:45, had warned us that we had to arrive on Staten Island and sit for two hours before the race began. If it was cold, as it should have been in New York in November, the wait would be brutal.

"I mean, I've got some stuff, but not too much," I said. "You know, if you're trying to run in three hours, we will not be running together, FYI."

"I'm probably going to get some extra warm clothes."

I did not normally run with a companion, so in the end, this turn of events was not terribly upsetting. We had been "training" together—me in Shelby Bottoms in East Nashville, Newt on a treadmill in a Manhattan apartment building—but the togetherness consisted primarily of periodic text-messaging more than anything. Needless to say, though, whatever deep confessions I may have been envisioning were clearly not going to happen. In hindsight, of course, I'm not sure we would have been able to hear very well at any point in the race, due to the cheering throngs that lined the course for the vast majority of the 26.2 miles, and after Mile Eighteen or so, there would not have been much coherence from me. But, for the record, Newt beat me by four minutes, and I ran it in 4:19:28, so he did not qualify for Boston.

After I crossed the finish line, I was extremely dizzy for a couple of minutes, but the race administrators wrapped me in a tin foil cape, gave me a goody bag of snacks, which I scarfed down in seconds, and herded me and many others through the park toward the exit on the west side. Because Greg lived on the east side, between First and Second Avenues, I actually had to walk through the park and five long blocks to his apartment. During this trek, ten or twelve random people on the street accosted me to wish me congratulations. I had families cheering me, one older man thanking me (I was wearing my charity shirt, so I suppose that's why I deserved thanks), a doorman at a building asking me how I had done (I told him, "I finished." He busted out laughing, as if what I said was exceedingly clever), and a twenty-something who was having beers with his friends outside giving me a shout-out. Finally, at one intersection, I overheard a little boy ask his dad if he could say something to me. His dad told him to go ahead. He very lightly pulled on my cape and told me, "Congratulations." I thanked him.

***

After the fifth IUI attempt failed, the TFC recommended we move to IVF (in-vitro fertilization). I remember that on our very first visit with the FD, IVF was discussed very briefly. It was a distant possibility at the time, something foreign in my mind—a last resort, moderately incomprehensible. It was, I thought, the "test-tube baby," the $20,000 investment, something that was extremely, unfathomably burdensome in all aspects. Clearly, I did not know much about it, and of course, I did no research on any medical endeavor of any kind. My wife, despite my entreaties otherwise, had been on the Internet nearly daily, developing a more extensive understanding of the process.

We had started to feel a certain amount of dissatisfaction with the TFC. Perhaps it was after a fifth IUI with absolutely no explanation for why things were not working or why throwing another $770.99 at this problem would accomplish anything the last four $770.99s had not. At this point, though, we were open to other options. And I, in particular, was ready to leave the TFC. I was done. The more we considered other alternatives, the more I stewed over the treatment and the TFC's train station-feel. The fact that the FD had raced through her explanations post-surgery became more galling. The fact that since that first meeting—in May—we had not had a thoughtful, fully-fleshed out sit-down with all three of us in the room to discuss our options and our course of treatment and the fact that we had simply been tossing pipettes full of semen at the problem became ridiculous. Why keep doing these? Why so casually tell us to just try it again?

Through the female grapevine we had learned some things: primarily that the TFC was essentially a monopoly in the area and that its success rate for IVF was fine, but nothing special. There were rumors about a good place in Atlanta. There was a renowned place in Colorado. We had no idea what we were getting into in terms of the time commitment, logistics, and the like for an IVF transfer and, perhaps, that is why we so willingly considered other cities. But I thought that if we were going to move forward with such a painstaking, difficult, and expensive endeavor, we wanted to do this only once: go to the best, go where we had the highest possibility of success.

At this time we heard from one of Julie's friends in New York about a Dallas endocrinologist and fertility specialist (hereinafter, the "Dallas Doctor" or the "DD"). The personal connection helped, and my wife had an initial series of phone calls with a woman at the DD's office who had had success via IVF with the Dallas Doctor and had positive things to say. His success rates (and these success rates are apparently externally regulated by an organization) were significantly higher than many others, including the TFC. The DD's office told us that the embryologist is the individual who really matters, and theirs was one of the best. Further, my wife had another close friend ("Q.") who lived in Dallas, and, thus, there was the possibility that Julie had a place to stay if she did undergo IVF down there. This option simply seemed to make a lot of sense. Quickly, we made the decision to try the doctor in Dallas. My wife flew down on November 14 and met with him for the first time. My uncle died the day before on November 13.

***

My uncle's death seems less enlightening to me than the others. It was not an unmitigated tragedy like David's death, but it was not a grandmother's death either, full and complete, after all that life had offered. It was a one-off death for me, experienced far more acutely by my cousins, my aunt, my mother. I had seen my uncle that one last time in September in good spirits at a celebration. I had not been there at the end, exhausted and devastated, watching it gradually and inevitably unfold—the man gone, his body still there, after a week of hospice.

In that way, I felt less of my own ego involved and instead, simply inadequacy, regret, and guilt maybe, that I was not going to be hit as hard, that it was significantly easier for me to move on, and that there was little that I could offer in support to anyone. We buzzed up there before his death, had a great weekend, partied, and enjoyed our time. We flew up there again for the funeral and partying seemed off; it seemed insufficient. The funeral felt insufficient. Leaving felt insufficient. Moving on so easily felt especially insufficient, knowing that others to whom I was close, would not and could not.

I had one story that I thought I could offer my cousin, Andrea, my uncle's oldest daughter, who was my age and had been a friend growing up. We had gone to a sports bar after the funeral with many family members and many Michigan friends, co-workers, and employees I did not know. The sports bar was in the midst of a typical Detroit suburb: commercial parks, upscale chains, nice strip malls sprinkled in with enormous, corporate headquarters. You could call it urban "sprawl," but if you just bounced from the sky into the airport, like we did, there seemed to be no origin, no beginning point from which all of this commerce and life had spread. And to the extent the center had not held, which it hadn't really,[47] and things had fallen apart, here, at least, the sprawl seemed to be doing OK. It was human development, human enterprise, and human pluck on a flat, cold landscape.

We sat at a long table at the sports bar. I was crammed on one side in a booth. At one point, Andrea sat down across from me.

"Oh, hey, how are you?" I said. I had not spoken to her much throughout the weekend, and I apparently had a tendency to revert to simple pleasantries when talking to someone when a tragedy was in the air.[48]

"I think I might be trapped in here," I said quickly. There was a pause. "You know I had a story about your dad. I should have told it." At the reception after the funeral, there had been one story told by the moderator with the microphone, but no one else had followed up. I was waiting on someone else to do something, and I thought that I would have been out of place, a random nephew.

"Oh, you should have," Andrea said.

"I know, it just, I don't know. You're right, though, I probably should have. It was one time when Uncle Bill was visiting New York City with Chloe (Andrea's younger sister, who had attended NYU), and we were out partying on Bleecker Street with some of my friends. Anyway, we somehow got onto a discussion about people who were too concerned with themselves, too self-

---

[47] See Chinua Achebe, *Things Fall Apart* (William Heinemann Ltd., 1958).

[48] After Greg called and told me David died, I volunteered to call another friend, Reed, because Greg didn't have his number. When I called Reed, he answered and said, "Hey, Stuart, what's up? How are you?" Out of habit, I responded, "Good, man," and then I stopped. "Actually, I'm sorry, not good at all…"

focused, depressed. Your dad expressed some impatience with those people and said something along the lines of, 'You know, in the beginning, why I went to work every day, why I got up every day, and why I did my job and have done so for years and years?'"

In this momentary break, someone close by who had been listening, started nodding and mouthed, "His kids."

I continued, "Well, yes, but not exactly. He said: 'Andrea.' He said that you, as a baby, were so cool, and your relationship through the years was so cool—that was the word he used: cool. And it was that connection and, of course, a similar connection with all of the rest of his kids, that made him get up, that drove him day-in and day-out."

I obviously didn't tell the story all that well, and it wasn't clear what, if anything, I had accomplished. Andrea had a blank look on her face—either she was touched and hearing that story was a good thing or it was too much at this particular point in time, or maybe it was just a little bit of an awkward story.

"You should have told that story at the reception," she said.

"I know, I'm sorry," I said. "I just wasn't sure." We were interrupted by someone wanting to speak to Andrea. She got up and left. The crowd, jammed in at this bar table, shifted. Before long, we went back to Bill's house with just the family.

In the end, maybe it wasn't that poignant, and so maybe I shouldn't have told it to anyone. Or maybe it just wasn't that big of a deal and what I said really didn't matter either way. What did I want? A fist-bump? I was a tourist popping in for a weekend and I had tossed out a story that, well, certainly didn't seem to sum up much of anything.

Dallas, Texas

"That was progress."

Assuming that I was able to meet a past version of myself—the version of myself that was lost on the fertility trail—and assuming that the two of us were able to suppress that inherent, human desire to beat the doppelgänger to death with Bamm-Bamm clubs,[49] what would we say? Could I use this interaction to make some sense of this experience? Because, right now, the thought of myself not so long ago seems foreign to me, and I'm left undertaking the difficult process of trying to reimagine myself during this time period: What was I thinking? How did we possibly do this? How did we function day-to-day with what was a continual, debilitating drain at the bottom of it all, gradually emptying out everything that was going on in our lives?

I can remember playing in a men's recreational soccer league in the midst of the fertility process. We played some of our games at a beautiful sports complex that Belmont University had renovated right in the middle of the Edgehill housing projects. I remember going to a few of these games at dusk. The field was built atop a random hill—one of seemingly few in Nashville— and I felt I was getting a rare glimpse above the fray of the valley below. This particular shot was of the Vanderbilt University hospital complex. On one particular evening, the sunset was remarkable, and I wondered if these sunsets happened like this every day up at a sports complex in the projects. But no one on the soccer team really knew me terribly well and obviously had no idea that, at that moment, I was in the process of struggling to have a baby.

---

[49] See *The Flintstones* (Hanna-Barbera, 1960-1966).

Apparently, it wasn't written on my face.

I can remember arriving at some of these games with such pent-up aggression, just a tangible frustration, both from our fertility struggles and probably just daily routine, working life, and I would be all hopped up, ready to get out there, roar like a wild animal, slam into somebody, and knock in a sixty-yard strike. Of course, most of that aggression was gone after about ten minutes of heavy sprinting. And slamming into anybody would probably have left me rolling around on the turf, fondly remembering that touching sunset I had just witnessed. But there was certainly a tangible sense of feeling sorry for myself, of wanting to go smash something or else go tackle that inflatable, West Virginia mascot and drool blood in his face like Brad Pitt on the mobster in *Fight Club*.[50]

More prosaic, of course, was what actually happened. I would willfully and knowingly head a goalie's sky-high punt. That's it. Usually in men's leagues, at my age, I and most other people with a brain will try to trap those punts that the goalie sends careening high into the air with a foot, not with the precious head. I can remember during these times damning it all to hell and going for those headers.

For my in-laws, I'm sure it was particularly difficult. They wouldn't see us day-to-day and thus, wouldn't see us when we managed to ignore the frustration for large periods of time, which was, in the end, how we functioned. Instead, they would only get calls from Julie where she'd be expressing the details of what was going on, and her anxiety and fears about the whole process, and there wasn't a whole lot they could do other than tell us to buck up and be patient and it'll work out. My father-in-law tells a story now and again of how Julie's younger sister Catherine called him from a pay phone one time while she was traveling abroad in France. She was crying and was going on and on about how they were stranded, and everyone was being rude to them, and no cab would pick them up, and they didn't know what to do, and they were carrying heavy backpacks, and it was raining, and it was all a horrible mess. I think he said at that point, "Catherine, I am on the other side of the ocean. I want to help you, but there is unfortunately absolutely nothing I can do. You are on your own, and you need to figure it out." I'm sure he felt something similar here.

For my family and, in particular, my mother and older sister, both of whom live in Nashville, this struggle manifested itself in a somewhat unexpected way, as fertility talk suddenly became a very normal thing. My

---

[50] *Fight Club* (Fox, 1999).

family doesn't share a ton of, you know, feelings or emotions or details of personal struggles and heartache. We, in general, prefer to analyze (and/or complain about) things. So it was a change, of course, to have my mother and sister versed in the ins-out-outs of the fertility process. There was no open questioning of it, no advice that I really needed to take a second, take a breath, re-think things for a moment, because my mother, in particular, is openly hands-off when it comes to decisions we make about our lives. Instead, it just became part of the day-to-day conversation: my mother, asking about an IUI. It was an issue neither of them ever had to deal with and probably had never seriously considered as something they would ever become familiar with, but I appreciated the fact that they took it in stride, treated it as a normal thing.

The IVF process, of course, ended up being more time-consuming for Julie than anybody. Her job, however, was very accommodating. Her immediate boss was a woman with kids and did not give her much, if any, push back. Her boss's boss has several daughters, and if anything ever came up where Julie had to ask him or tell him about an upcoming absence, he'd give her a, "Do what you need to do," before she even got close to explaining what was going on.

My job is flexible with time off, but I can remember telling one of the assistants in our office that I had to go to Dallas mid-week for a few days.

"For something fun, I hope," she said.

I responded, "No, I wish."

"Work?" she asked.

"No, not really work, either, but definitely not something fun." I left it at that.

Otherwise, day-to-day, strangely, my relationship with Julie seemed to improve. I had certainly heard, and now have heard more, tales from friends that fertility struggles caused divisions in their marriage—that these particular difficulties promoted discord. For us, although my narrative, at times, may seem to indicate otherwise, it was actually quite the opposite. I have been told, on occasion, that I am a naturally self-centered person. (I like to say "introvert.") During this time, however, things improved on that front. I would anticipate things that needed doing around the house. I would volunteer to help out when Julie had something she needed to do. If Julie mentioned something to me that I found completely irrational, instead of immediately discarding the idea or arguing on behalf of myself, I'd take a second and think about her and where she was coming from before I responded. It was all very new and different.

I think I took to having something specific to do, to focus on, a clear way to help out. Or maybe this ever-present struggle that we were both experiencing forced me to be less self-focused and more empathetic. In fact, perhaps I took to it because it actually involved simultaneously both empathy and self-focus, because this was something we both were suffering through. A self-focused empathy—now that is an empathy I can get interested in! Whatever it was, throughout this process, I was allegedly a better husband than I have ever been, before or since.

***

The night cloaked the city like a blanket. As I remember it, while learning similes and metaphors in grade school, this was the workbook, simile example, the quintessence of simile, timeless and classic: The night cloaked the city like a warm and fuzzy blanket. How's this for a modern and almost assuredly immediately outdated simile: My memory of our first IVF experience in Dallas and everything that goes with it meanders in my mind like the Apple TV screen saver set to "Floating." I thought screen savers were long outdated here in the early 2010s—the bouncing, morphing, iridescent orb on the old Windows computers has been replaced with a plain, quiet-time, black-screen, sleep mode and, even wandering around my office at work, the only other alternatives, the only screen savers I meet on rare occasions are scrolling quotes—"Travel with a candle, instead of a flashlight"—and nothing else, no changing landscapes or geodesic designs.

Apple TV, however, still utilizes the old-school, hard-freaking-core screen saver. When you leave it sitting for more than five minutes, the photos come up, Apple TV-robot-randomly-chosen from any and all pictures that have been transferred from my phone or camera to my computer over the past few years, different trips, different Instagrammed shots. They mosey on by, each fully contained in and of itself, and yet completely unconnected to the others. So it was with this trip to Dallas.

The memories haphazardly drift, mere flashes rather than fully-fleshed-out experiences: too many care packages from my wife's friends, piled on top of one another, enough books to read for months; a discussion of a basketball team; a phone call with the doctor from our kitchen table in Nashville with hastily sketched out notes; the births of good friends' babies; Texas road construction; and, of course, syringes, syringes large and small, syringes for mixing, syringes for shooting, trigger syringes, bruised backsides, vials of clear liquid, and my searching, always searching, for bare, fresh skin to jam one in.

And so I will try to access these moments in a coherent fashion. Like Data playing for the tie[51] or, else, like the Super Mario Brothers 3-playing, wizard boy,[52] I hope to sit down, jiggle a few buttons, discover the warp zone, wopp-wopp down, and make this happen.

***

In making sense of our seven-month TFC run, there was a clearly discernible transition that occurred. Let's call it "the quiet dissipation of hope." Up until the laparoscopy, there was always a feeling that we had just not adequately addressed the problem. As such, our attempts had no chance at all to work, so in essence, we had no hope in what we were doing. After the surgery, however, the surgery that supposedly fixed the most likely cause of the infertility, and the fifty-day or so wait in between periods that accompanied the surgery, we believed that we had made progress and that now our attempts were worthwhile. We were at least playing on an endometriosis-less playing field. That is, someone had finally gotten up, grabbed a few friends, and lugged the goals that had been sitting upside down on the sidelines out onto the field.

The TFC's and the entire "fertility" process's approach to the problem is certainly an attempt to assert control over what is usually an all-natural, uncontrollable human process. For an IUI: force ovulation, ensure that an egg has been produced, make the egg drop, insert swimmers directly into the uterus and then leave things up to the great overlord in the sky. (IVF takes it a few steps further.) It's a wrestling back of control over a process that you wouldn't think, or never did think, needed such micromanagement.

This belief that you can control each aspect of this process certainly has a psychological impact. Thus, during our time at the TFC, we kept trying to exert just a tad bit more control over what was going on. At one point, in the midst of our slew of IUIs, it appeared that we may have been timing the IUI incorrectly so that my wife would get a shot, and according to something we had read or heard somewhere, we should have been having the IUI an exact amount of time after the shot, thirty-six hours precisely. The way the TFC had scheduled us seemed not as exact as it could have been, and our thought was that those few hours one way or the other could make all the difference (in the world!) and would be the opening, the quiet sliver that we needed to finally break through.

During one of the IUIs, Julie raised this issue with the FD and instead of

---

[51] See "Peak Performance," *Star Trek: The Next Generation* (Paramount, July 10, 1989).
[52] See *The Wizard* (Universal, 1989).

being shot down or dismissed out of hand as the wondering of a worrisome woman, the FD or the nurse or whoever was present actually responded with an audible, "Oh, yeah, maybe we *should* do it that way."

Afterward, when I was being told this story, I said, "So they said they should have been doing it that way all along?"

"I mean," she said, "that's what it sounded like."

I was perturbed, "Is that a joke?" I waited a second. "Who is running the show over there? Why are we telling them what needs to be done?"

"Stuart," she responded, "I really don't know; that's just what she said."

It was as if they hadn't already thought of that, or else they might have been doing it wrong and not even worrying about it, as they made us go through another one of these Opryland Barnstormer airplane rides— around and around and around, tied down—without even making sure that everything was properly in place.

Of course, maybe they were humoring us and they knew that it did not matter one way or the other. And maybe there are limits to the amount of control anyone can exert over this process (short of creating your own embryos). Under the circumstances, though, I thought we either could in some ways control it, in which case we should try to control as many aspects as possible, or we could not actually control it. Success or failure should not hinge on random suggestions from the patient.

Or maybe people need to take responsibility for their own health care. Then again, we were paying for expertise, I thought, even when the process was not necessarily ingenious, not necessarily, breathtakingly brilliant like the Dyson bathroom hand dryer. Let's pay them $700 to inject sperm all up in there instead of letting the good old-fashioned penis do it! Even if that is the case, though, please do something, expert; tell us something; at the least, be in charge. And if the exact hours matter, let's adjust our schedules accordingly. If the hours don't matter, tell us they don't matter. Don't pretend that they do matter and that we just came up with a brilliant new idea simply by reading the Internet.

In the end, this dissipation of hope wears. And the fifth time around we were not starting out with much hope to begin with, so that when it started to dissipate, it disappeared fast, like water on grass rather than frost on glass.

Further, as each subsequent IUI ticked by, it appeared that we were being outsourced to an underling, where a nurse, at best, would take my wife's calls about our next IUI. Perhaps she was reporting directly to our FD, but either way, it appeared all she was getting back was a recommendation to try yet another IUI. I can imagine how this conversation went—in the TFC's bustling hallway, the FD late, rushing by, the nurse or other orderly, nervous, mentioning my wife's name, the FD thinking for a split second before making a few connections and then saying, "another IUI," as she walked into another room for another examination, another IUI, another consultation where she might recommend an IUI to whomever might walk in.

Even beyond this lack of a genuine leader in charge of our regimen—our fertility trail guide—other frustrations abounded. I know there are plenty of clichés out there waiting to be uttered by mankind,[53] and here I am happy to oblige. One of these is that, "you just know," you know? Wait, you don't know? That is, "you just know if you're pregnant." With these IUIs, we were obviously never provided that moment, but we were also never even given the opportunity for the other clichéd experience of waiting and wishing and hoping, while a pregnancy test worked its urine-interpreting-tea-leaves magic and the two of us clutched one another in blissful anticipation. For us, the IUIs never got that far.

I feel that men encounter hope in our daily lives most often in a rather acute, albeit entirely meaningless, manner: sports. We subconsciously may intuit that anything that happens to whatever team we root for actually does not make a single shit bit of difference in our daily lives, but there is, at the same time, a certain amount of legitimate investment. For instance, while watching your football team attempt to come from behind at the end of the game, there is a certain amount of hope—perhaps irrational if you've been following the Titans in the post-Steve McNair era—that your quarterback just might be able to put a few things together and somehow miraculously engineer a victory. (Full tilt on clichés.)

When that doesn't happen and your hopes are "dashed" and the ball tumbles to the turf and undergoes a few awkward, dead-fish flopping bounces before the piano explodes,[54] there is a tangible sense of hope lost, of all that adrenaline rushing from your body and mind, when you realize your quarterback just threw an interception. Or else, it was fourth and fifteen, and you knew that he was going to get sacked and/or throw up a pass that would

---

[53] The writing process feels, at times, like being Pac-Man: constantly moving, gobbling up the facts, spilling out a story through round, easy-to-see, little pellets, but always having to avoid the clichés, which may arrive in various colors but always in the same shape, floating along lightly, gliding, trying to interrupt. Thus, I feel myself stopping abruptly, moving in the other direction, jerking around in a geometric U-turn, slipping out one side tunnel into the brief unknown before back quickly again, forever doing what I can to dodge the clichés, which forever appear anywhere and always. I wonder sometimes how I speak, how I communicate without them.

[54] See Faith No More, "Epic" (Slash/Reprise, 1990).

have no opportunity whatsoever to be caught. As you helplessly watch, there is the immediate, visceral feeling of failure. It can be tough to deal with at the moment, depending on your level of disillusionment. You might want to take a bat and smash it over someone else's lawn furniture, or, if you are wearied and worn out with your team, you might be able to write it off and file it away as just another broken promise, Bud![55] But there is a moment where hope existed followed by one in which that hope suddenly and completely disappeared.

Here, that never happened. We were never afforded that sorry recompense, that moment where we could pinpoint Ralphie's heart ripping in half,[56] where we realized that, despite our best efforts, we had not been successful and had lost.

Instead, a day or two or three or a week after the actual IUI, one morning I would wake up to discover that Julie was already out of bed. I could see a light on in the bathroom. It was early, and day had not yet dawned. She had said a few times since this particular IUI and once the night before that "I don't think it worked. I just don't feel any different." I usually didn't respond to these comments. I couldn't tell her she did feel differently. I thought it better, under the circumstances, to simply try to ignore what she was saying.

The room felt empty. I knew she was using one of the pregnancy tests. [$30 apiece.] My impression, though, was that she was trying to rush it, that she wanted to try one out even before the doctor had recommended it, so even though we were pretty sure it had not worked, we could at least pretend to have that moment of a clear-cut answer, that moment where hope existed.

The light would go off, and she would quietly come back to bed. I could tell by her face or by her walk, even in the darkness, even without putting my glasses on, that she was pretending that she wasn't surprised or disappointed. That she had expected that particular answer. She'd slide back into bed, and we'd pretend to sleep. And so, failure gradually became present—something that had always been standing there that I just happened to notice.

***

In early October after the Femara rounds continued to fail, Julie made the decision to switch her OB/GYN. At that time, it was my impression that we had next-to-no relationship with OB1 after she referred us to the TFC,

---

[55] Bud Adams, Houston Oilers/Tennessee Titans owner from the team's inception in or around 1959 to his death in 2013.

[56] See "I Love Lisa," *The Simpsons* (Fox, 1993).

but my wife, of course, had had at least a few interactions of which I was not aware and had perhaps felt a disconnect, so that a change seemed preferable.

Our new OB/GYN ("OB2") tested Julie's Vitamin D levels as recently news of the importance of this particular vitamin to one's overall health had been slithering up in various places. My wife was also tested for the Cystic Fibrosis gene. [Covered by insurance.] She tested negative, but OB2 did find that Julie's Vitamin D levels were extremely low, somewhere around sixteen where "normal" is considered between thirty and eighty. OB2 put her on a prescription strength dose of Vitamin D—a 50,000 IU pill to be taken once a week for one year. [Covered by insurance.] Other than that, she encouraged my wife to be patient, not to be discouraged, and not to be too paranoid about the endometriosis. OB2 said she had personally delivered many babies to women with endometriosis, often untreated endometriosis found during a C-section.

Further, as noted above, we had made the decision to move forward with the Dallas Doctor, the DD. During my wife's first trip down there, the November 14 appointment, the DD did a routine exam followed by a vaginal ultrasound. Based on the findings from the ultrasound, he felt that once and for all, the PCOS diagnosis was incorrect. He said he did find small cysts on my wife's ovaries, but that there were not enough to deem them polycystic. He also walked Julie through several scenarios of seemingly healthy people who could not get pregnant (and then succeeded in getting pregnant under his care). The majority of their problems ended up being immunological, and he mentioned how he was an advocate of immunological testing to diagnose specific fertility issues.

He said this was a bit controversial—or, at least, that not all fertility doctors placed as much importance on these immune disorders—but in his experience they had proved significant. He also performed more tests on Julie's thyroid and endocrine system, claiming too many fertility doctors placed too much importance on the obstetric/gynecological side of getting pregnant and not the endocrinological. At his urging, we had the immunological testing done, called the Repeated Pregnancy Loss Panel. [$2,976 for consultation and testing.]

On December 3, we received a letter from the DD outlining his findings. He said my wife's TSH (thyroid) was slightly elevated at "3.84." He wanted her to begin taking 50mcg of Synthroid to suppress her thyroid, as he wanted it at or below "2.5" as we tried to conceive. They also found her "natural killer cell activation activity was remarkably high at 13.9 percent where normal is less than ten percent." (The explanation we got for the "natural killer cells" phenomenon was never crystal clear, but the gist was that a high level of natural killer cells can create an environment where natural killer cells attack healthy embryos before they can implant—a problem that would obviously interfere with fertilization.) He then recommended "a cycle of in vitro fertilization embryo transfer with intralipid being given prior to embryo transfer to suppress natural killer cell activation."

As you might imagine, a new approach sounded great to us, especially from a doctor who wanted to address the problem from a different perspective. For me, at the time—and now—it made loads more sense to research and attempt to diagnose a problem first rather than attempting a solution without ever figuring out how bad the problem was.

We discovered there were two schools of thought in fertility. The first is advocated by those with a strictly OB/GYN background who push for tries, tries, tries: This is the way babies are made, so let's keep throwing it up there and one of these is sure to go in. The second is advocated by those who study and are assumedly experts in hormones: If the baby-making is not working naturally or not working via IUIs, perhaps fixing a hormone problem in the woman will or could make normal baby-making more successful. Implicit in this second school of thought is the idea—perhaps never actually vocalized, but definitely there—that if the hormone problem was fixed, then normal, good old-fashioned, stick-it-in-there baby-making might work. While this ultimate solution may have been implied, it was still seemingly always under the guise of an IVF recommendation: We'll fix your hormone problem, but you'll still need IVF.

But this made sense to me: sperm and egg wasn't working. Let's look at the egg production facility and figure out if we can fix a few things there that might allow sperm and egg to better connect. Further, this "natural killer cell" business sounded as good an explanation as any that had sidled up to the bar throughout this process. It definitely appeared to be something I could latch onto, a legitimate answer. Plus the treatment for natural killer cell activation sounded fairly innocuous. An "intralipid" was an infusion of fat, just good old-fashioned fat that would essentially distract natural killer cell activity or suppress it in some capacity. It sounded easy, straight-forward, simple, yet brilliant.

So, yes, we were drinking the Texas Kool-Aid. When you were where we were, though, knowing that IVF was more than likely going to be the next step, we wanted to do it somewhere that would give us hope of success, which was something the TFC could no longer provide. Otherwise, we would what? Stop everything and forget it? Think about adoption?

For whatever reason, outwardly expressed or not, adoption always seemed to be something to consider after IVF. Because really, that could not be the way it worked: a bunch of IUIs, lorded over by a distracted FD, and then it's over and you adopt? That was not a good enough shot. Plus, these seemed to be two fundamentally different, yet equally wrenching and difficult processes: Either commit yourself to the fertility process and believe that it is going to work or commit yourself to adoption. It wasn't quite possible just to jump to the other so readily.

Actually, the more relevant concern, at this point, was not adoption, but the fact that any discussion of IVF included a serious discussion of the possibility of *twins*. I entertained this idea in an abstract way. I certainly said the words, talked about it, expressed wonder and confusion at the possibility. I heard about others with twins. At the time, though, that seemed, simply, a bridge that we would happily drive our moving van[57] across if the fertility trail ever led up to its rickety, insane planks.

* * *

The IVF process was going to begin in January 2012 once my wife got her period and would last six to eight weeks into mid-February, depending on how quickly her eggs grew. Julie got her period on January 3 and started taking birth control pills at that time. These were used to regulate her cycle and ensure that she would begin taking Lupron (see below) at the proper time. It also prevented ovarian cyst formation. We both started taking an antibiotic, Doxycycline, on January 5 and took it for ten days.

Julie and I also both went to a chain medical lab on January 6 to get a battery of tests done. They included (for her): FSH, Hepatitis B antibodies, LH, Prolactin, Rubella, Estradiol, blood type and blood RH type, Hepatitis C antibodies, viral antibodies, and TSH. I had all of the same Hepatitis tests, HIV, and maybe a few others, but to be honest, I wasn't paying attention.

Obviously, a medical lab was not somewhere I would choose to spend a morning, a weekday breakfast out with my wife. Then again, at this point, it's not even worth noting that this was an inconvenience or that this sucked and annoyed me, and I should have been at work drafting motions. In the grand story, this was such a minor blip, such an inconsequential occurrence that, in hindsight, it was actually somewhat surprising how efficient the whole thing was.

---

[57] See *Funny Farm* (Warner Bros., 1988).

The lab was notable, though, in that this place is full of highly toxic, contagious, deadly diseases and crazily potent drugs. But, oh yeah, it's run by a couple of nurses, one of whom pissed the other one off by being late to work and who looked like she might have had a late night, by which I mean, of course, that she may have gotten drunk the night before. And now she was jumping into her routine—without thinking, it seemed—of tying off my arm and sticking me with a needle to draw blood, pack it up, and send it off somewhere to some other hungover twenty-year-old to be tested for highly communicable diseases.

I suppose in any situation like this involving modern health care, there is a certain necessary suspension of disbelief of the Shakespearean variety. The idea is that when watching a play, although you understand that everything up on stage is pure artifice, in order to be entertained, you dive into the fiction for a little while, imagining that everything is real. Here, it was similar: Everything I saw convinced me that this whole process was fake, a joke, completely "make-believe." That is, I didn't believe for a second that this woman was going to properly draw this blood, package it, and successfully send it off, and I doubted that anyone in some lab in Atlanta was actually going to get it and properly test it for anything without screwing something up royally. At the same time, in order to do what needed to be done, I disregarded all the little details in front of me and trusted that it was real and that everything was actually functioning as it was supposed to.

I do think that, unless you happen to be a medical professional, you need to have some of this blind trust in any medical situation. Certainly, you can be ultra-paranoid, which is not totally irrational after any number of recent medical fiascos, which would seem to call this artifice to the surface. But unless you are fully committed and ready and willing to go all-natural and refuse vaccines for your child, then some trust seems to be necessary. Here, I was happy to have blood drawn and then get out of there. Of course, my poor wife had to sit through longer draws, further tests, and multiple hours in the medical equivalent of a McDonald's while I scurried on to work.[58]

---

[58] It's worth mentioning that we received a bill from the lab, many months later in December 2012 for this lab work. We, of course, thought we had already paid this bill, and thus we had to make a few calls to Dallas and to the lab to figure this all out and ensure it had been paid appropriately. We had, indeed, already paid it, but then again, if I didn't get a bill for a medical procedure performed that I had already paid for or my insurance was supposed to pay for and did not, I might forget for a moment that I was in America.

***

A few weeks later, on January 18, Julie flew back to Dallas for a "trial transfer" and IVF class.

IVF consists of two major steps: the "retrieval" of eggs from the woman and the "transfer" of an embryo into the woman. In between these two procedures, the embryologist takes eggs and sperm in a lab, gets them to mate, and then hopes that they will turn into little embryos, as many as possible based on the number of eggs "retrieved," or, as my older sister kept saying not entirely inaccurately, "extracted." (Retrieval calls to mind a mom in a sundress beckoning the kids for dinner—extraction, a tooth being ripped out.)

Along the way, some eggs don't mate with the sperm sample, some eggs don't make it at all because they are too weak, and so, even if you retrieve a large number of eggs, only a certain percentage may end up creating embryos. Those embryos are grown in a *Matrix* field of humans, harvested by evil robots,[59] or actually, no need to be negative, let's say, a magic garden somewhere, a field of flowers, harvested by Barbaloots frisking about in their Barbaloot suits,[60] before two are then implanted, or "transferred," from the field of barley to the woman's uterus, where we all hope at least one of them "takes" and grows into a fetus.

At the trial transfer, the DD did another vaginal ultrasound to measure my wife's uterus (this had to be performed on a specific date, around the time she would normally be ovulating), so that he knew the most optimal place to position the embryos on her actual transfer day. They then walked Julie through all of the medications she would be taking, how to give herself the shots, how to order the medication, and the payment schedule. At that visit we paid for the trial transfer and class, plus all of the lab work that had been performed. [$1,650 for fertility clinic activities, plus one-way ticket to Dallas: $140.30 (we used points for the other leg).]

At the time, I can remember the Dallas Doctor's office was a bit confused as to why I was not accompanying my wife in for the trial transfer and class. There seemed to be a communication breakdown between whomever was running our fertility plan, presumably a nurse, and the woman at the front desk, presumably a scrivener, who was handling logistics. On a few different occasions it became clear that this doctor did not have a ton of out-of-town patients. That is completely understandable as retrieval to transfer

---

[59] See *The Matrix* (Warner Bros., 1999).

[60] See Dr. Seuss, *The Lorax* (Random House, 1971).

is a multi-week process, and IVF is a physically, emotionally, mentally, and psychologically draining experience, and trying to do it while living nine hours away seemed to be the height of boneheadedness. At the same time, we were also under the impression that this DD was one of the best in all the land and had one of the highest success rates in the country, and thus, he did have experience with out-of-towners. Having to clue the woman on the phone in on multiple occasions that we did not live in Dallas was a tad disconcerting. But it's just something we ignored, and in general, at this point on the fertility trail, you have to ignore a number of such details.

After informing whomever that I was not coming in and after a few discussions, phone calls, and consultations, it was determined that they might need me to provide a semen sample and then FedEx it to Dallas. Apparently, at a trial transfer, the man typically provides a "specimen,"[61] so that on the day of the retrieval, if, for some strange reason, he cannot perform, they would have a cryo-preserved cup of jizz on-hand to make the magic happen. That made sense, so with my wife bartering communication between a handful of different actors, we managed to order semen-shipping packaging that arrived at our house. At one particular lunchtime, I raced my car home, had a party, followed the directions, filled up a little cylinder, threw Nordic ice packs in there, and then swung by the FedEx Office on my way back to work. [$78.93 for FedEx; $175 for the packaging.] I can't imagine that the FedEx woman possibly knew what it was, but she seemed to give me a knowing glance and was polite and discreet.

***

On January 18 while in Dallas, my wife began her first medication, Lupron. Lupron prevents the woman from having a luteinizing hormone surge, which happens when a woman is about to ovulate. In short, it's a drug that *suppresses* ovulation, so that the woman does not ovulate before the doctor has determined that the follicles are ready.

The Lupron was one of the easier shots. It was smaller and taken in the stomach—about two inches or so, as the crow flies, southeast or-west of the navel. Typically, the shot-giver, which was usually me, although Julie certainly had to give herself a good many of these on her own, would pinch a bit of the skin in the stomach, alcohol-swab it, and then casually slide the little needle in. Unlike others that would come later, this was a casual injection, not a poke;

---

[61] *SpeciMEN*, early potential book title.

if you poked, you usually drew blood and garnered a physical cringe from the patient. Instead, the proper way would be for the patient to pinch the skin and look away while you, the shot-giver, should just move it on into the skin at a steady, consistent pace, shoot the trigger of the syringe, and it's over. Once you get used to the aggressive jab in the backside, coming back to the Lupron can be tough, as you may have trepidation that you have lost that steady hand. Be not afraid. Be confident.

At first, it seems pretty rough to be shooting anyone, let alone your wife, in the tenderness of the stomach, but when all is said and done, you will look back and think that the Lupron shot was nothing. Julie was injected with Lupron once a day for fourteen days.

Around February 3, we started the Menopur shots. Menopur shots are notable for their name, which was definitely the coolest of any of the fertility drugs, as it called to mind bad, sci-fi movie superdrugs that the entire population would take and turn into beautiful drones. It contained FSH and LH. According to one information sheet we received, it is "used at various points of the cycle when determined by your doctor." On the outside of the vial, it says, "trust me" on one side and "inject me" on the other.[62]

It also involved "mixing." I had not, up until this experience, given a lot of shots to anyone. Mixing certainly sounded daunting to me, but we thought, if it's too terribly complicated, I'm sure they would not let normal peons do it at home with no experience, no training, and just a website to check for proper instruction.

On the appointed day, we attempted our first Menopur shot. Our computer was open on the counter in our kitchen. We pushed aside the kitchen clutter and cleared out room to work. We had been instructed to watch an Internet video instructing how exactly to go about conducting the "mixing." We pressed play.

We never saw the face of the woman in the video—just a backside and midriff. The voice told us that one vial had powder in it. We found the powder vial. With one syringe we were supposed to extract purified water—no, sorry, make that "diluent" (pronounced as it is spelled—DILL-U-ENT). "Diluent" is a word you may not hear much in your life if you aren't in the medical profession, but when you're trying to figure out how to give a Menopur shot, you're going to hear "diluent" about fifteen times per minute, a freak hail storm of "diluents," before hopefully, it fades from your life as quickly as it came—from a different vial, and then inject it into the small vial of powder. I think I

---

[62] See Lewis Carroll, *Alice's Adventures in Wonderland* (Macmillan, 1865).

did this. I was then supposed to mix in a swirling motion—not shaking, but swirling or whirling—until the powder disappeared. Again, as instructed, I whirled. At this point, I was to switch needle tops on the syringe, extract a certain portion of the mixed liquid, and then inject.

"They don't tell you how to change the needle," I said.

"Where's the other needle top?" she asked.

"How does it say you're supposed to switch the needle tops? She just has a new one," I responded. I was mumbling. "Hers looks different than ours." "Her" being the woman in the video.

"Oh, wait, hold on. I mean, it looks like the powder has disappeared."

"All right, all right. I got it. It's supposed to, though, right?"

"Is that too much?" she asked. Things were getting out of hand.

"Probably," I said.

"Wait—what did you just do?"

"I don't know; I thought I put it back." The kitchen began tilting in space.

"That's the diluent."

"Fuck." Disaster.

It sounds, in hindsight, relatively straightforward. But, as you might expect, when attempting to follow directions in an anal-retentive manner by doing exactly what that midriff-baring woman was saying at every point in time, I found myself tripping up, or else staying too tied to the mechanisms of the process and not letting the natural artistry of shot-giving come into play. If I had been more comfortable with it, with the tools, perhaps it would have been an easier process.

As it were, somehow on our first shot, we (or I) managed to screw it up. The diluent vial and the powder vial somehow both ended up having the mixture in them at some level or another, so that we lost track of how much diluent had been injected into how much powder and then they all were mixed together and somehow transported back into a different vial and the woman was deaf to our pleas and one of the needle tops she was using was slightly different than the ones we were using, so maybe that was it?

We discarded one set of vials [$4.50], tried again, and as far as we knew, were successful.

Julie also started taking 225 IUs of Gonal-f once a day, along with periodic Menopur, while the Lupron was still going strong. Gonal-f is a follicle-stimulating hormone that stimulates the ovaries to grow follicles. Gonal-f was, again, a mixture, but a more simplified one as all the diluent went straight into the powder, and then you extracted the entire amount of Gonal-f for injection. This still involved all injections in the stomach area, "subcutaneous," although the needles for the Gonal-f were slightly bigger than the tiny, sweet, little girl Lupron needles.

Once you start doubling up shots, you have to switch from one side to the other: right side in the morning, left side in the evening. When you go back to the right side on the following morning, you obviously try to avoid the spot from the morning before. You continue dancing around each morning and evening until you have a field to work with—a speckled array of little pinpricks. At that point, on occasion, you might vary noticeably lower or to the west or east on a whim, here and there, but you'll inevitably come back to the compact field of landmines. [Drug charges around this time: $91.80 + $2,867.08 + $129.]

Maybe the shots, physically, were a bit like baby showers emotionally: just so intense, so painful that there was not really a whole lot that I could do in support. As noted above, throughout our fertility experience, my particular way of approaching my relationship with Julie had gotten discernibly better. In hindsight, though, I'm thinking that I probably didn't transform all that much, maybe it was just logical: I was jabbing my wife with large needles, morning and night, while at the same time I knew that this whole process, while difficult at times for me, was far more emotionally wrenching for her on an every-waking-moment basis. Thus, suddenly, my initial, ingrained reaction to defend myself at all costs seemed less important. How would it make sense to argue with someone whom I had just had to poke with a giant needle? And not just one needle, one time; I just had to pick out a good spot that did not already have a needle mark scar on her stomach, of all places, or her backside, and then stab her again. And she did it without ever really complaining. So, maybe, my inclination to be nice was just a reflection of my admiration for Julie and her toughness.

***

At this point, I still had maintained a certain amount of reticence about going into this topic with friends and, at best, had been cryptic about the whole thing. Leading up to the Dallas experience, we had been given a tip sheet of things that I, the man, needed to do in preparation, including cutting down on booze, refraining from wearing tight pants, and—no joke—icing down my testicles each night. (The woman's tip sheet was more like an owner's manual.) This wasn't anything specific to me, personally, just the typical handout given to men in order to try to maximize sperm count. I was not in any position to ever stop wearing skin-tight pants, but cutting back on booze seemed reasonable.

About that time, my friend Peter invited me to a Nashville Predators hockey game with a few others. I declined with a strange e-mail response, where I said I had "personal things going on, namely, Julie will be undergoing a semi-major medical procedure here in about six weeks, with which I am involved...if that makes sense." I rambled on for a bit longer about "embarking on this thing" and how my wife was nervous, etc. No details, just purposeful, incomprehensibly vague gibberish. Alternatively, I could have responded, "Can't make it, bros, bummer!" and left it at that, but clearly I was trying to reach out in some very limited capacity.

Later, a phone conversation randomly occurred with my friend Taylor where I talked, again, rather obliquely about how "this" was all happening in Dallas, how we had chosen to go to Dallas because they had much better success rates, and we had been majorly frustrated with the whole process in Nashville. He sounded interested and certainly did not have a whole lot of understanding as to what I was talking about, or how it all worked, or why a trip to Dallas was necessary, but again, I left it at that. My cagey responses would have given anyone the feeling that they shouldn't ask about it unless I chose to bring it up.

Much later, after our fertility experience had ended, I was at a wedding in Philadelphia where the wife of one of my college friends was about to undergo an IVF transfer back in Virginia, while he was at the wedding. He talked openly, knowingly, and in detail all about what was happening, in the presence of several of my other friends, including Taylor, as if they inherently knew the terminology and/or the process.

"It's intense, you know. At this point, I've given her so many shots I can't even look at a needle—I just tell her, you gotta do it." We were eating croque monsieurs at a French bistro in downtown Philadelphia.

"If this doesn't work, I don't even fucking know. Man, the people I've seen in some fertility clinics at 7:00 a.m. are some interesting-looking people." A grizzled veteran, I stared at an object in the surroundings and kept quiet.

"She called last night while we were out. I missed about six calls—now she won't answer. I think they should be transferring embryos as we speak."

Taylor shook his head at the moderately ridiculous, hungover Saturday morning, embryo commentary. My single friend wasn't paying attention. It was probably up for debate whether anyone was comfortable talking about all of it in such a public forum.

But is it something that even needs to be publicly discussed? Should people be comfortable with it? It obviously pales in seriousness to something like, say, Alzheimer's disease, that would certainly benefit from being more comfortably discussed in public so that people—both outsiders and those affected by it—understand that it's a disease, like any other and thus, not anything to be embarrassed about. Alzheimer's just so happens to make the victims of the disease do horribly embarrassing things that they would never otherwise do. Obviously, traveling the fertility trail is not anywhere close to the same planet as the experience for all involved of a harpy disease like Alzheimer's that snatches the victim's brain and changes his personality and leaves him living—because, honestly, that's some real sci-fi, *Fringe* shit,[63] and the center really cannot hold, when there's personality-changing diseases on the loose—but, at the same time, I certainly don't think infertility should be handled in a slapdash, ham-fisted, completely unserious way either. Like, say, Liz Lemon jokingly having "trouble" in the final season of *30 Rock*, half-assingly giving herself fertility shots, apparently injecting herself with hormones for a couple of days for fun.[64] Not to sound like an old woman's blouse,[65] but I have to say I was disappointed at how that was dealt with, because haphazardly shooting yourself with drugs for a while before deciding to adopt is not actually how it works. And I'm not trying to be a grown man who still breastfeeds, but give me a fucking break. It's not like that at all. It sucks. The whole process sucks. Maybe everyone doesn't need to understand it, wear ribbons for people who are struggling with it, or understand the details of all that goes into the long and trying ordeal, but they also don't need a poorly sketched out, slapdick version of the experience that makes it seem like a laugh that can be cured with an, "Oh, hey, yeah, why don't you just adopt?"

Also around this time, some of my good friends' babies started being born. I felt no resentment, no envy at all, but these were not friends who lived in Nashville, so in many different connotations, I was worlds away. So I just sent a text maybe. It was simply not something with which I was involved.

***

It all began. Around this time, late January to early February, Julie was having ultrasounds performed at the TFC [\$230 + \$95 each time (x 4) = \$1300] to monitor the follicle growth. They sent the results to Dallas, and the DD would alter my wife's drug dosage accordingly. On Friday, February

---

[63] See *Fringe* (Fox, 2008-2013).

[64] "Game Over," *30 Rock* (Universal, Jan. 10, 2013).

[65] See Mr. Bates, *Downton Abbey* (Carnival Films, 2010-present).

10, Julie flew to Dallas [$130.30] for the duration. The DD performed an ultrasound himself that afternoon to decide when the retrieval should take place. He then had her come back in on Sunday to check on the follicle growth again. My wife stayed with her friend Q., who took over the shots at this time.

The DD decided that we were probably going to trigger Monday night, February 13, and have the retrieval on Wednesday, February 15. The plan was for me to drive to Dallas on Sunday morning to be there for the trigger and the retrieval, and then fly back to Nashville Wednesday night, because, after the retrieval, there would be almost five days before the transfer.

Thus, we finally make it to General Nathan Bedford Forrest. What a relief. As a Nashvillian and long-native Tennessean—my dad's roots, on one line, run way, way back, a-drop-of-Creek-blood back (although, technically, that's south Georgia rather than Tennessee, but southern nonetheless, 1600s-Creek-blood-southern) and, as far as Nashville goes, I'm a fourth generation Vanderbilt graduate, also on my dad's side—it is, I feel, worthwhile to have some basic understanding of Nathan Bedford Forrest, who, along with Andrew Jackson, is probably the most famous/infamous of Tennessee's historical figures.

There is a clownish statue of Forrest surrounded by rebel flags out I-65 South near Brentwood, just south of Nashville, which caused a stir when it was erected at some point in my adolescence, and it apparently still stirs up forceful feelings even now, as does Forrest himself. Of course, the statue itself is so bogus, with a cartoon grin, that I imagine the man himself would have torn it down with his bare hands and eaten it if he had known it existed.

I had done research on Forrest for a college paper while at the University of Nottingham for an art history class called Visualizing War (when you say it in your mind, please use a ridiculous, college-professor-inflected British accent for the "War," i.e. "Woor"). The professor was a caricature of flimsiness who canceled three of nine classes because he was "sick" and had a tendency to note, in an attempt to foster discussion, that a painting was "BIZZAH." Discuss.

I used a portrait, a daguerreotype of Forrest, all stern eyebrows, gaunt face; white, flowing, crazed hair, to make a point on how we understand images. When I presented to the class, I noted that the British students probably didn't know much of a half-dead chicken (an old southern saying, I said) about the American Civil War. But, if I were to tell you that it was rumored General Forrest never lost a battle he was in (not entirely true, but mostly true and part of the legend), and that, although backwoods and country (born in Bedford County, Tennessee, about an hour southeast of Nashville), with no formal education, he had a brilliant military mind (very true), you would think one thing. If I told you he was the first Grand Wizard of the Ku Klux Klan, your opinion and, by extension, this portrait would change. Deep stuff.

In my effort to expand my knowledge of this backyard, historical figure, I found what turned out to be a fabulous biography of Forrest[66] and bought the audio version in anticipation of my drive. Thus, on Sunday morning, I slurped a big cup of coffee at home, and knowing I didn't need any more coffee but unable to help myself, I filled up a to-go cup, hopped in the car bright and early in the seven a.m. range, popped in the Forrest bio, and screamed out of Nashville, high on life and hope. The IVF process had finally begun. It was a necessary process, it was something we had chosen to embark on, it was something to which we were committed, and it was going to work.

I was jammin' through Memphis, over the Mississippi, and into Arkansas as the tale of Forrest evolved over the airwaves. The coffee was still going strong—whooooweee was it going strong—and I was thinking, man oh man, a pre-war Memphis would be a fascinating setting for an HBO drama: a major, slave-trading port, by lantern light, mud and blood in the streets. Or, if we went blockbuster, Colin Farrell to play Forrest. Yes! Oh, the trailer, at the very least, would be amazing and, you know, full of exploding lanterns. Boom! In fact, there would be so many exploding lanterns in the trailer I just don't even know what to do. F-O-R-R-E-S-T ticking across the screen at the end. Shazzam!

As the coffee subsided, I continued on through Arkansas with Little Rock off on the right, the one pop-up of civilization in a bare stretch of American interstate, eight lanes of shimmering cement,[67] before Texarkana and east Texas with its giant, right-wing, political positions pasted on billboards against an otherwise flat and featureless landscape. Finally, Dallas appeared on the horizon, fifty miles away, a vast metropolis beyond a lake, as interstates started circling, swirling, half-piping above and around as I sped into town. I arrived at Q's house in Dallas.

* * *

On Monday, February 13, 2012, I accompanied my wife to the DD's office for another ultrasound that would confirm that we were going to trigger that night. The "trigger" was an intra-muscular shot that would force the follicles to drop. This shot had to be taken at 9:00 p.m. on the dot. The eggs then "drop"

---

66 Jack Hurst, *Nathan Bedford Forrest* (Vintage, 1993).
67 See *Who Framed Roger Rabbit?* (Touchstone Pictures, 1988).

exactly thirty-six hours later, when the DD would be there to retrieve them.[68]

Thus, I took my first trip to the DD. The DD's office was in a high-rise connected with the Baylor University hospital system. There was a massive amount of construction in and around the office, and my car either needed new shocks or the metal slabs we were driving over were many inches thick, because traveling to the office involved a notable amount of bouncing over construction materials. In general, these details are not something one thinks too much about except when you happen to be anticipating that you will later be driving around with a woman who has just been injected with embryos, and you don't want them to bounce right out, so it was slightly more of a concern. But that was to come. Here, we were in for just another doctor's visit.

The office was old-fashioned, at least in terms of wall art, which I was comfortable with and recognized well. My father, when he was practicing, had a remarkable collection of old paintings of owls lining the halls in his office. It had a slight tinge of the country doctor feel, which at the moment, I preferred far more to the TFC's Penn Station-vibe.

The DD was an older doctor with certain older-man mannerisms, a peculiar way of speaking being the most notable. If you had him on the phone and had never met him, his slow-motion tone and frequent, long pauses, might be disconcerting—as if he were confused or even elderly—and you would be hesitant to invest your anticipated future children into his care. When you met him, you certainly understood that he was not confused or elderly, but smart and clearly possessing an ample amount of knowledge about what he was doing. He also had a wry, dry, or completely desiccated sense of humor and a peculiar manner of explaining medical issues to patients through joke and convoluted anecdote. I remember two particular comments he made on my first visit. One was allaying certain fears about multiples.

My wife asked, "Do you ever consider transferring more than two embryos?"

He responded, "No, we don't want a basketball team." Basketball? Oh, a starting five, right. OK.

---

[68] At some point in my life, I happened upon a nasty, interstate, gas station bathroom where some lost and clever soul had scratched graffiti into the hand dryer. Usually, toilet graffiti in such decrepit spaces causes one to question the existence of humanity's soul, but here someone had scratched in some interesting, hand-dryer commentary. The symbols instructing one how to use a hand-dryer have the warm air pictured as red squiggly lines of what apparently (to someone) looks like bacon. The strange mind had noted that when drying one's hands, one retrieves bacon. You make bacon by pressing the button, then you retrieve bacon. Scratching that missive into a hand-dryer had to have taken some time, so graffitist friend, learn now, it was worth it.

And second, in discussions of the natural killer cell diagnosis, he told a story of an Indian woman who had had multiple miscarriages over many years. "She would be several months pregnant each time, and she'd lose the baby again and again and again," he said. A brief pause. "And then, she came to me, and we treated the natural killer cells." Pause. "She had a healthy baby. So I don't really know what to say, but it seemed to do something for her."

"What a great story,[69]" I thought. To be honest, though, that wasn't exactly the explanation that I was looking for: "It seemed to work for someone else one time, so there's got to be something to it…and, oh yeah, be thankful you haven't had a bunch of miscarriages thus far."

Again, when dealing with a medical professional, especially this far into the process, there was nothing we could do—ask for a new doctor?—and, as I had done so many times before, I just laughed it off. I thought that there must be more to this diagnosis and procedure than that. He was clearly just trying to highlight a point that, sometimes, the solution may be straightforward. After months and months or years and years of trying, you may ultimately discover that one primary issue was causing your problem, and, after a quick antidote, all would be better. But still, this story did not provide much reassurance, and I knew exactly what Julie was going to think the minute this story concluded: Oh no, I am in store for many miscarriages in the years to come.

Then again, perhaps his explanation about the Indian woman was slightly more honest from a fertility doctor's perspective. She was having trouble; we tried something different; it worked. That's how the whole process works. No one has any idea and, if someone could actually guarantee a result, needless to say, they'd be very successful. Sure, yeah, some guesses have proven to be more successful *on average* than others, so we'll keep trying those to see if we can get anything to work. But realize, everyone, that this process is still one giant, uncertain guess. We couldn't dwell on these details though. We were already aboard whatever flying umbrella[70] we were on, and it certainly was not going to change at this point.

Or maybe, as my wife said later, he was just cocky. With his meandering way of speaking, I certainly did not pick up on it, but she may have been right. Trust me, he was saying, I've fixed far worse situations than yours. As I said, his success rate was significantly higher than the TFC and anything we had heard about elsewhere. Obviously, he probably had smaller sample sizes than these bigger shops, but assumedly the numbers don't lie. [Bills paid to the Dallas

---

[69] See *Parenthood* (Imagine Entertainment, 1989).

[70] See *Robin Hood* (Disney, 1973).

office around this time: $486 + $685; drug company: $145.80.]

**

It was confirmed at this visit that the trigger shot would be given that night at 9:00 p.m. At that point, we had not given any shots intramuscularly (in the backside), so the nurses at the office gave me a tutorial. We sat in a conference room, while two nurses stood above me, bandying needles about. "When giving all shots," one of them, a wiry woman about our age from Texarkana, said, "you pull back the trigger to bring a little bit of air into the empty syringe, and then inject that air into the vial, before pulling back whatever is in the vial into the syringe. Then you tap the syringe to get whatever air bubbles happen to be in the syringe to rise to the top. You try to eject those little bubbles by squirting out a bit of the liquid, shaking the dew off the lily, and then you're ready to go." (For the record, I'm pretty sure she did not actually use the phrase "shaking the dew off the lily.")

The nurses then showed me how to inject the trigger syringe, which was exactly like the progesterone shots to come, all of which go in the right or left buttocks. My wife would pull her pants down about halfway, a fair amount of room to work with. I'd alcohol up the entry point, the target area, a few inches below the hip and to the right or left, closer to the outside of the leg, and then *Pulp Fiction* it straight in with one fluid motion.[71] The most important thing for this shot was that you came in with enough force that the needle went all the way in. Once it was in, you injected the liquid. If you came in limp-wristed, soggy-handing it, you might only get the needle halfway in. Then you'd have to provide a second, awkward shiv-jab at which point you could feel the needle slowly sliding through muscle, which was bad.

There was a certain amount of pressure for this trigger shot. We had to get it right, directly at 9:00 p.m., and having no prior experience with the intramuscular injections, we were nervous. But, as I said before, I'm my own effing man. My wife stood in Q.'s kitchen ready to be frisked, and the trigger shot went right in. No problem. And when you're able to pull it off, with no blood whatsoever popping back in the needle, you know it's been a perfect pour.

The next day was Valentine's Day, and my wife and I went to see *The Vow* at a swanky Highland Park movie theater.[72] Julie was shocked at the time that

---

[71] See *Pulp Fiction* (Miramax, 1994).
[72] *The Vow* (Spyglass, 2012).

I would so willingly agree to see such a pointless movie. But I thought that I certainly owed her far more than one screening of a romantic comedy.[73]

***

The Retrieval: The DD's office occupied half of a floor in the office building. The other half was a surgical facility, and the two sides connected through an emergency, swinging door. We proceeded from the country doctor's office to your more typical hospital room, where nurses prepped Julie for the procedure. We sat in freezing cold temperatures while a little box TV of morning talk shows hung on the wall. I provided my sample (see Hustler-Vivid porno discussion above), and she received anesthesia from a man wearing a gold chain with exposed chest hair who looked like he was from New Jersey. But he was extremely friendly and seemed thoughtful and concerned about his patient, so even if he had looked like Lil' V, playing with his own shit in the shower, I would have been fine with it.[74]

Eventually, my wife was wheeled to the surgical room. I covered myself in an extra sheet and tried to keep my eyes open, as we had been up since 5:30 a.m. I had some coffee that morning, but because I had not waited a sufficient number of days after the road-trip coffee, the alertness and the sustained, wonderfully jittery buzz that it would have provided if I had given it a good two-day break was not there. Instead, it made me a little cracked-out, but mostly drowsy, so I hunched and periodically checked my phone while I tried

---

[73] For a number of different reasons, the first of which, of course, was the fertility treatments she was being subjected to. Secondly, I thought I probably owed her at least, let's say, twenty or so *Vows*, after some of the movies I had forced her to see, in the theater, over the years. The most egregious that come to mind and, for vastly different reasons, are *Willard* (New Line, 2003), *Ponyo* (Disney, 2008), and *Enter the Void* (Wild Bunch, 2010).

[74] Actually, scratch that, I would not have been fine with our anesthesiologist playing with his own shit. On that note, I'm not saying I care much of a hoot to even discuss the matter and I know *The Sopranos* had started a perpetual, downward plummet far before the scene with Lil' V playing with his shit in the shower, but I'm not sure any show has crystallized its own moment of abject, disgusting failure, than the scene with Lil' V playing with his shit. See "Chasing It," *The Sopranos* (HBO, 2007). *Lost* might have had the most devastatingly awful final season, the most depressing of all total catastrophes, when the curtain was pulled aside and instead of a brilliant master plan of invention and mystique and a floating green cloud of awesomeness, there were simply two dudes sitting in fold-out chairs, jerking off. But, at least on screen, *Lost* never had a moment where new Chinese guy with baseball was caught in the temple playing with his own shit quite like Lil' V's playing with his own shit in the shower. See *Lost* (Bad Robot Productions, 2004-2010).

and failed to doze.

The process was not terribly long and soon swinging doors were flying open, nurses were steering her back in, and doctors were slapping each other on the back, laughing about another conversation. Julie was coming out of a daze as we heard about the number of eggs retrieved: sixteen! Sixteen is a very high number, but when they told us, Julie appeared openly disappointed. The doctors saw this and laughed heartily again.

The reason she was disappointed was because that morning Julie continued to ask questions in hopes of relieving certain fears. In response to these questions, the doctor decided to tell us a new story. You see, he had had one particular patient, who actually had twenty-four eggs, but those eggs ended up only producing two embryos, while another patient had only four eggs but produced one good embryo, which developed into a pregnancy. "One is all you need," he said. I understood his point, of course, but I also understood my wife's immediate, visceral reaction to that story: risk. There was a risk we could produce fifty eggs and get zero embryos, so even with sixteen eggs, nothing was guaranteed just yet.

Maybe it's a generational thing or an old, white, male, OB/GYN thing,[75] but fertility doctors clearly do not have any sense of the actual experience of meeting with a fertility doctor. They do not realize how challenging this process is. If they did, they would provide definite answers and otherwise speak in platitudes: "This is your problem. That is it. We will fix it. Everything is going to be fine. This is going to work." Facts about the randomness of it all do not help. Stories about women who have multiple miscarriages do not help. Talking about women having five babies also does not help.

The anesthesiologist returned to check on her soon thereafter. Julie was high on drugs and got into a loud conversation with the doctor about his daughter, who apparently attended the University of Indiana. I was generally under the impression that my wife knew next to nothing about the University of Indiana or the state of Indiana, but she spoke, quite loudly and proudly and sincerely—"That is such a great school! I'm so happy for her."—as if she herself were a recent alumna. She was just trying to be nice, of course, and the doctor knew it and reciprocated. After that, we stayed a little while as the drugs wore off. With the help of one of the nurses, we wheeled Julie down to the basement parking garage and headed back to Q.'s house. [$5,070.]

---

[75] Another one of my maternal uncles mentioned a story at a holiday recently of his early experience in medical training in Chattanooga and how an old, white man OB/GYN, who had been around forever, used to joke, while sewing up a woman after she had given birth, that he would make it just the right size to fit him, the doctor.

When we arrived at Q.'s house, I was sent to Walgreens to pick up an antibiotic and estrogen patches. [$53.93 + another bill for $64.23 a few days later.] I received a free *Dallas Morning News* upon entering the store, although I had to inform the nice lady that I lived in Nashville, and it was highly unlikely that I was going to start a subscription. She looked sad. I ordered the prescription, waited in the car, and read the paper as the pharmacists counted their beans in the back—hockey, I believe, was most interesting to me. I then returned to Q.'s house.

I had transported on my drive a number of frozen Tupperware containers full of homemade chicken noodle soup that my wife had made before she flew to Dallas. I attempted to heat one of these in a pan, when it should have naturally gone in a microwave. I proceeded to burn the bottom of the pan and reduce the chicken noodle soup to chicken noodle pasta. I could hear someone in the next room and I felt a fool. I took the dish up to my wife, and she appeared deeply annoyed. She seemed to toss the bowl aside, as if I *was* a fool and didn't know how to boil an egg. I knew it was the anesthesia talking, but there was something about feeding my poor wife after she had gone through yet another ridiculous medical procedure that usually provided me with solace. But that afternoon, she wasn't having it. Then again, she was more than likely subconsciously annoyed that I was scheduled to fly out *that evening*.

Before I did, we applied the estrogen patches, which looked just like nicotine patches. We were supposed to load up with about five or so across her lower abdomen. The nurses had also recommended an ointment, Goo Gone basically, which would get rid of the residue when they were removed.

I also gave her the first progesterone shot—a shot that, in hindsight, is truly the only one that springs to mind when I think about this process. It was basically identical to the trigger shot: a big honking needle, right in the backside. I did not know at the time that it was the first of very, very, very many to come. (Think two times per day, moving forward, from here on out, through the rest of this story: every day, one shot in the morning and one shot at night, unless I tell you otherwise.) I jabbed her once. She got in bed. I said a quick good-bye, tried to compensate with a longer-than-usual hug, and I was off, back home to Nashville. [$130.20 for one-way flight.]

***

Our grand plan was that, after the retrieval on Wednesday, my wife would have five days off until the transfer on Monday, February 20. During this five-day span, the eggs were fertilized, and the embryos were grown. (On February 17, two days following the retrieval, Julie had an intralipid infusion, i.e. the treatment for the abnormally high number of natural killer cells. [$188 + $91.80 to drug company.])

The retrieval involved anesthesia as the procedure was more of a medical one, while the transfer itself was simply an injection. Although she may have been given a Valium or the like, it was not as invasive. So we figured it made more sense for me to be there for the retrieval as I could take her to the hospital, be with her throughout the process, and take care of her a bit (or for one afternoon) afterward. Because the transfer took only a couple of hours, she could simply get a ride to the hospital and back. After that, she would be on bed rest for three days, so it didn't make too much sense for me to be simply hanging about all that time.

In hindsight, this was terribly wrong. Yes, it was useful to have me there, driving Julie to the hospital and helping her into the car afterward, but psychologically, the retrieval was over and successful the moment my wife came out of anesthesia. We knew that it had worked and that they had been able to retrieve plenty of eggs to work with. The transfer, on the other hand, although less physically trying, packed an emotional and psychological wallop that neither of us was anticipating: They are in there! This is the pivotal moment! Let's hope it takes! Oh yeah, sit around for three days and don't worry about it.

During this five-day break before the transfer, I was at home, going to work, acting like a normal person. On Saturday night, I stumbled onto *Paranormal Activity* on Netflix and watched both the first and second versions[76] by myself. I talked to Julie in the middle of one of them, and she and Q. were both shocked that I was watching these movies at home, in an empty house, at night, in the dark. Q. was in the room with her during this conversation, so we did not really delve into much. Julie sounded in high spirits.

She did not tell me on this call or any of the others we had during this stretch, but instead, long afterward, that the aftermath of the retrieval was far more physically painful than expected. Since she had the laparoscopy only several months earlier, they said her midsection was probably still a bit tender. As such, the pain lasted several days.

The error in our planning, however, did not become glaringly apparent until a few days later, on February 20, the morning of the scheduled transfer.

---

[76] *Paranormal Activity* (Paramount, 2009); *Paranormal Activity 2* (Paramount, 2010).

I was at work again when she called, and, again, I got up and closed my door.

"Hey," I said.

"Hey," Julie said. "We are at this furniture store, and they have a very good deal on this ottoman for the end of our bed. What do you think?"

"An ottoman?" I said.

"Yeah, I think it goes perfectly with our bedspread. It's a good deal, but it's not going to be available for very long. I think it would definitely fit in my car. What do you think?"

"Wait, where are you?" I was confused. I was under the impression that the transfer was supposed to take place, basically, at any moment.

"We're at a store right near Q's house. We really need something for that room," she said.

"Aren't you scheduled to have, you know, a transfer, like, right now?" I said.

"What?" she said. It was difficult to hear. "I bet you don't care. I don't know why I called you. You can't make a decision about anything."

That made me perturbed. "What are you talking about? A decision on the ottoman?"

"Yes, the ottoman," she said. "That's what I am talking about."

"Yeah," I responded, "I don't give a shit about the ottoman. Get the fucking ottoman. I don't care. I mean, what are you all doing? Aren't you supposed to be at the hospital right now?"

I was sufficiently worked up at this point and rude, and I think she hung up on me. In hindsight, if I could have ignored my self-focused indignation at being yelled at over a footstool, I might have been able to see that my wife was hurting and was royally freaked out. And I was sitting in front of my computer, in Nashville, doing legal work. Instead, we bickered on the phone for a bit, and then she was gone.

She told me afterward that Q. had dropped her off at the doctor's office, and Julie called her fifteen minutes later in tears. Q. returned and stayed with her throughout the transfer.

We also thought that my sitting around while she was on bed rest would not be a terribly valuable use of my time. If she was just going to be watching movies and reading books (and she had ample books to read, enough care packages from friends and family members to stave off boredom in a bomb shelter for at least the first few months of a zombie apocalypse) and she was at Q's house and would have someone to bring her lunch and periodically keep her company, what good would I do?

As it actually worked out, though, on Day Two of bed rest, I got another call:

"This is infuriating," she said.

"What is it?" I asked. I was, of course, staring at a computer screen. Getting calls out of the blue from an infuriated wife, when she was supposed to be on bed rest, calm and serene, was a little jarring, although I tried to respond this time in a more positive manner.

"I mean, I've called the DD's office three times now, and I can't get anyone to call me back."

"For what?" I asked.

"I'm trying to set up the second intralipid infusion, and they've got nobody they can recommend in Nashville. OB2 has no idea what this is, and she can't give it. I just don't know who else I'm supposed to call."

I paused. Did I have any idea where to look for this? "They don't have any name for anyone in Nashville? I mean, I would think they would know somebody."

"No," she said. "And right now the nurse won't call me back. There's some dialysis center that does it, but they won't administer the procedure for fertility purposes. I've already left three messages."

"Well, I mean, you really don't need to be worrying about this or dealing with this right now." That was obvious, although I went ahead and said it anyway.

"I know."

I sympathized, of course, but there was only so much I could do over the phone to help, to ease her from flights of fancy, albeit rational ones. I could have taken over the burden of tracking this information down, but at the time, she had a far better handle on it and I had been, and still was, outsourcing most of the logistics to her.

I imagine on that day of rest she probably spent much of it in bed on the Internet, fretting that we would not find someone in time, and everything we had just done would all be for naught because we couldn't figure out some basic details. Eventually, she tracked down a Walgreens affiliated with Vanderbilt that would offer it at their minute clinic and got it figured out.

I flew back to Dallas on Thursday night. Q's husband picked me up at the airport, and my wife took her first trip downstairs in three days for take-out in front of the television. The next morning after a quick trip to pick up our new ottoman, we drove the nine hours back to Nashville.

At one point during dinner in front of the TV that night, Julie made a comment along the lines of, "I'm sure, knowing my luck, we're going to end up with twins," with the implication that we better get used to the craziness that that would involve. I can remember my thought was that we should probably just take one step at a time. One step. First and foremost, let's get a positive pregnancy test. At the time, though, I kept my mouth shut.

**

After the retrieval, the embryologist had performed ICSI (intracytoplasmic sperm injection) on the eggs, manually fertilizing them with the sperm, after which we all waited to see how many grew at a favorable rate. The embryologist tracked the progress of the embryos daily and would call Julie with updates. Over the weekend, before the Monday transfer, he called to say that seven were growing at a favorable rate.

They ended up transferring two embryos. We came to find out later that these two were at the "morula" stage and not the blastocyst stage, and the blastocyst stage is apparently preferred.[77] After transferring two, we waited to see what happened with the other five. They do not like to freeze embryos unless they are blastocysts as they are more likely to "take" if they are further progressed. They called Julie the following day, Day Six after retrieval, to tell her they wanted to wait to watch their growth an additional day before freezing them. At this point, they were down to four embryos, as two had been implanted and one had trailed off. We learned afterward that 95 percent of embryos reach the blastocyst stage by Day Six, and ours had not. On Day Seven they had all reached the blastocyst or "extended" blastocyst stage, meaning they were in the process of hatching, and they froze all four. They told us that all would be viable for future transfers.

**

We were back in Nashville by Friday night, February 25. On the following Wednesday, February 29, we had our first pregnancy test. We scored a six. I did not know what that meant.

I do not remember the phone call with Julie when she communicated to me that we had scored a six on a "levels of pregnancy" chart that I heretofore did not know existed. This particular memory is simply not there. Maybe it was because I was not being told anything acute, clear-cut, or plain: an obvious answer, an obvious failure, an "it did not work." Perhaps it was because I believed the old saying that you're either pregnant or you're not, and, if we were pregnant, I was looking for a plus sign and celebration to ensue from

---

[77] FYI: Zygote → Morula → Blastocyst.

all around. Thus, when I was informed that, first, they forgot to mention that there is a new scale we need to become familiar with, the HCG scale, and it's going to measure just how pregnant we really are; and, second, the new scale we just discovered says that one through five is not pregnant and we scored a six, it simply did not compute. As such, nothing about this moment comes to mind.

The pregnancy tests measure HCG (human chorionic gonadotropin—the hormone produced by the placenta when a woman becomes pregnant), and the powers that be wanted to see a level above five. We scored a six, which was, in my mind, above five. Earlier that day, Julie had a pregnancy blood test performed at OB2's office. OB2's office then faxed the results to the DD. The DD, however, was out of the country, and it took his office most of the day to get back to us. Which left us waiting for someone, somewhere, to clue us in. When they finally did call, the people in Dallas told Julie that they usually see it around thirty plus at that point or, at the least, fifteen, so six was not good.

The DD communicated from overseas, though, that there was still hope, that Julie should get another test on Friday, and that there was a chance the embryo/s was/were simply taking their time. Because we were higher than a five, they kept Julie on the progesterone shots and the estrogen patches, and scheduled another test two days later on March 2. We had hope, right? The doctor said so.

Later Wednesday, though, my wife had a quick discussion with a woman in the DD's office, the one who had originally helped recruit us to the DD. She told it to her straight that it was highly unlikely that she was pregnant (or Julie had probably gotten "pregnant" but immediately miscarried). So we shouldn't have had any hope whatsoever.

My wife was filling me in on all of these details, but, as I mentioned, these moments are simply not there. I do not purport to have much Funes[78] in me—that is, full, complete, all-consuming recall—but, in general, I usually have some recollection of where I was and what I was experiencing at certain pivotal moments in my life; but here, there is nothing.

I do remember that my father-in-law called me at work, late in the day, soon after we concluded that we were basically not pregnant. He and Julie's stepmother had been planning to come to town from Roanoke that weekend, and he wanted to get my thoughts on whether that was still something they should do.

I saw his number on my phone. I stood up, closed the door to my office.

---

[78] See Jorge Luis Borges, "Funes the Memorious" (Editorial Sur, 1942).

I was somber, I remember that, and I said, "Of course. Believe me, Julie would certainly want you here and, I mean, we both would want you all here regardless."

"Well," he responded, "I just didn't know if this was something…that maybe you all just needed to spend some time alone together. I know this has been hard on both of you."

"No, I mean, this has definitely been far worse on Julie," I said. "But, honestly, we have spent plenty of time together, you know, talking and thinking about this," I winced. "At this point, any kind of support…" I paused. I could feel myself grimacing. I put my hands on my head, fingers on my forehead.

"Well, I thought, at the very least," he said, "I could just give my little girl a hug."

My voice was strained, "Yes, yes, I would appreciate that."

I said that even if this didn't work, which it doesn't look like it had, I didn't think, it would be better to have them here than not here. If by some miracle, it did end up working, then obviously we could celebrate.

***

I never thought of myself as an overly hopeful person and really I'm not, but I do trust in other people and trust that, in most situations, people are going to do their jobs and do them correctly. Thus, later that night in bed, rationalizing out loud to Julie, I said, "Look, they would not keep you on these hormones if there was no chance whatsoever. If this expert doctor and his years of experience think that we may still have a shot, then we might as well hope that we still do or pretend that we still do."

"OK," she responded. She didn't argue.

There was simply not a whole lot else we could do, obviously. If we were going to keep taking the drugs and the DD said there was a possibility, we had to believe that something might happen.

On Friday, something did. Julie went back into OB2's office for the follow-up pregnancy test. This time, OB2's office simply called her directly. She scored a twenty-six.

I would be lying if I said I was not significantly heartened by the twenty-six—pumped, actually. I do remember that conversation and, again, I was at my desk in my office underground. I didn't stand up; I stayed in my chair with a computer screen blazing in front of me. I stared past the screen at the beige, scuffed wall, where a power cord sprouted plug buds. Ready to launch into telephone condolences, I was shocked. A twenty-six? A reprieve? I was reserved, certainly, rationally, not letting myself go entirely, but because the six had been next-to-nothing, the twenty-six had to be something, right? We were way above five now. Had to be pregnant. Plus, quadrupling! What else could the DD possibly have been looking for?

I e-mailed my mother and my older sister after this second test. I remember the excitement of sending that e-mail and dropping crazy-positive news on them out of their computer screens:

> So she goes back in today, and the pregnancy hormone is at twenty-six, which is really high (the doctor was looking for the number to double; it has quadrupled…I think this is a good thing). All in all, she hasn't had a phone call with the doctor, so we don't really know what this means. It still might go back down, she still might not be pregnant. I, a. don't really believe that it has worked, and/or b. am probably naturally putting up defense mechanisms so as not to be too devastated again if it turns out not to be happening, but, regardless, better news today than we have had before.

A bizarre hailstorm swept through our neighborhood in the midst of all of this on Friday afternoon. My wife sought cover in a parking garage at the Green Hills Mall while talking to the DD's nurse at the time. I was at home with my iPhone, recording the golf-ball hail bouncing off our back porch. Julie's dad and stepmom had pulled over on I-40, thirty minutes outside of town.

When they arrived, we told them the news. Twenty-six, bam! We were still restrained, of course, but twenty-six!

I know we grasped that hope on Friday and then tried to self-consciously forget about it. We tried to go through the weekend as if it were a normal one—we weren't dwelling, staring at a phone, at a stove clock, at a watch, waiting for time to progress and the pregnancy to take. We were consciously and deliberately trying not to talk or think about it.

For some reason, though, inevitably, relentlessly, doubt settled in. It just started to feel more and more likely that we were fooling ourselves. We were simply pretending. I started to feel something similar to what we had experienced during our many IUIs, although more acute. In just a day or two, as the weekend fell away, I started to anticipate that we were going to look up on Monday, like a Lotus-Eater,[79] and discover that it was over, and that

---

[79] See Homer, *The Odyssey* (8th Century B.C.).

we weren't even there to see it end. This hope was flimsy; it could be brushed aside by a night or two of sleep.

While going through the weekend, we kept up positive appearances. But when we were back in the bedroom, at night or in the morning, before venturing out to visit with the family and make coffee and skim the Sunday edition of the *Tennessean*, I could tell by looking at Julie. This isn't what it was supposed to be like. If the cliché is that "you just know," then we knew.

After the weekend with my in-laws, Julie went back in on Monday. Given that three days had passed, apparently the HCG level should have more than doubled. It was forty-seven. So it had increased, but not doubled. (Then again, forty-seven isn't that far from fifty-two, right? Am I missing something?) We were told on Monday that the chances were essentially less than one percent that the pregnancy would be viable. Even with this supreme unlikelihood, though, they still decided to keep her on the progesterone and estrogen. She had to go in again on Thursday, three days later, for one more test.

I do remember these calls. Maybe so many occurred while I was at work that they simply have been fused together and notable distinctions have faded. I saw my phone buzz. I got up and shut the door again. While shutting the door, I answered and then, more than likely, paced in my office. Or sat, facing the wall.

"It didn't work," she said.

"OK, love. We figured as much at this point," I responded. "I'm really sorry."

"*I'm* sorry." She was crying.

"You, obviously, don't need to apologize for anything. This is just…this is bad, but we'll get through it."

My wife's level was down to fifteen at the next test, so she was allowed to stop the progesterone and estrogen at that point, so the pregnancy would naturally pass on its own. A few days later, she had her period.

I know that afterward, months later, my wife would refer to this experience as a pregnancy: a pregnancy, and a miscarriage. I would bristle ever-so-slightly. Technically, I thought it was a "chemical pregnancy" rather than a miscarriage. But perhaps this was and is something for women and not something about which a man should express any opinion or thought whatsoever. But, in my mind at least, this was not a pregnancy. There was no miscarriage. That's not how it works. Not that it matters, but I think it's important to be clear that this was not a success in any way. If we accomplished nothing on this trip, let us be damn sure, that in whatever rates of success calculus that governs the work of fertility doctors, and in particular, that number that the DD had that was significantly higher than the national average, let us be sure that this particular IVF goes in the record books as a 100 percent failure—not a pregnancy and then a miscarriage; a total failure.

After the final test on Thursday, we had a call scheduled with the DD on Saturday.

***

We were emotionally wiped out at this point and, yes, it was a roller coaster. Although roller coasters are all about thrill and reprieve, thrill and reprieve, or perhaps constant thrill, swinging around a corner, plummeting down a ravine. This experience was more blind, wishful hope, followed by confusion, temporary despair, alleviated by a sudden break with the attendant, not-entirely-blind, but optimistic hope, followed by chunks of that hope getting lopped off, day-to-day, hour-to-hour, a lump at a time, until whatever form that hope was in collapsed into nothing. So I guess it actually wasn't like a fucking roller coaster at all.

Even though now I may seem filled with righteous indignation and misplaced bluster, at the time of our call with the DD, we were not in the mood to be angry or dissatisfied or to point fingers. We simply, still, after all of this time, wanted an explanation, an answer. Why didn't it work?

For the phone call, I attempted to take the lead as Julie did not want to and we agreed that it would not make a ton of sense for her to do so anyway. We had a list of questions to ask, and I attempted to take copious notes.

He was heartened that the pregnancy tried to take. We expressed a lot of concern about the quality of the embryos given their slower growth rate. The DD was adamant that it was not an issue and that was not necessarily an indicator of embryo health as embryos grow at different rates in different ways. Even though the embryologist had told us that ours grew slower than ninety-five percent of the healthy embryos they see, the DD said that because ours continued to evolve and their growth didn't arrest this was positive.

His take was that the HCG levels had started out lower, which is generally not a good sign but is not necessarily one hundred percent conclusive. In the end, though, he said the pregnancy must have had a genetic, chromosomal defect. The body simply did not allow it to progress and that it happens in a good many cases.

I thought at the time and again, afterward, when my wife would recite this explanation to whomever—her parents, my parents, her close friends—that the "chromosomal" defect discussion lacked certain qualities indicative of good, strong language. Namely, it did not communicate its point well. Because when I heard that, I thought that our sperm and egg had combined to create a monster, and the body had killed it off. Likewise, this thought coupled with another: that there was something about our fundamental genetics, our combined DNA, which made them simply not compatible. Either way, I didn't know if that was indeed what happened or not, but I knew it did no good to try to dwell on that. I've had a lot of explanations for this entire experience, for the inability to make work *the* fundamental human process, but I'll gladly take PCOS or polyps or endometriosis or Vitamin D deficiency or natural killer cells over "genetic abnormality" any time.

Plus, the question inevitably arose in my mind: How often in our previous experiences with the IUIs, and even before, did we have a microscope and recording device this early in the process? In a normal situation, without all of the test tubes and drugs, she would have simply had what we thought was a heavy period, period. There would have been no tracking, no 6-26-47-15. It would have been: No, no pregnancy, it didn't work, so there would have been nothing to be "positive" about. How many of these could have happened in the past? Perhaps, we were getting pregnant, but nothing was ever taking. Is that what inherent chromosomal defects would cause?

We asked about the natural killer cells, and about how maybe there had not been enough of the intralipid infusion, or we hadn't done it soon enough afterward. He said that the one infusion lowers the level of natural killer cells in almost everyone and that for the majority of women one infusion is enough. He said, in the future, we could possibly have an infusion the minute after we had a positive pregnancy test, but that suggestion more than anything seemed to be an attempt to humor us.

Otherwise, there was some confusion. The doctor's notes said something about the shells around the eggs being thicker than normal. The doctor had another anecdote about one woman, one patient who had strangely thick eggshells, so the embryo simply couldn't hatch. He thought ours may have been thicker than average. But my wife spoke to the embryologist later who said that the eggshells on the embryos were fine, not abnormal.

We asked the DD, what would the process be if we were going to try this again? How soon could we go? He was supportive in our moving forward with a frozen embryo transfer after the next cycle.

Finally, he noted that it was his intuition that "we will have a child," based on his having done this thousands of times, and that, in the end, this experience, although disappointing, was positive: We had had a pregnancy. That was progress.

Medieval Times Parking Lot, Dallas

"No, I was happy."

"I don't know if this is even an appropriate question at this point, but, I mean, do you even want to have a baby?" Newt asked.

"Yes, Newt," I responded. "At this point, yes, I do."

Newt had taken most of my tale about our fertility struggles in stride—that is, he did not seem terribly shocked. As I might have guessed, he said his wife and Julie had perhaps discussed the matter briefly recently, so he was not completely unaware. Plus, I'm sure he probably knew someone else who had dealt with this at some point, and so maybe what I thought was this totally unique experience of ours was not unheard of. Maybe, in fact, plenty of people know about the basics of what is involved. What I was happy about, though, is that he didn't give me an "Oh, it'll work eventually," or an "I'm sure everything is going to be fine." Instead, he just listened.

"How's your dad doing?" Newt asked. I had done a very good job up until this point of never telling any of my friends much of anything about our fertility struggles. Julie, however, had not allowed that to happen with the news about my father. Instead, without any explicit go-ahead from me, she reached out to several of them and told them that my dad had been diagnosed with Alzheimer's disease. She usually knew best in such situations.

"Hey, man, thanks for asking," I responded. "He's doing OK. He's basically plateaued—in a good way. He bikes three or four times a week, sometimes, like, seventy to a hundred miles a day."

"Oh, wow."

"He keeps himself busy. I think he's enjoying his retirement in a way," I said. "And, honestly, with all of this fertility business going on, it's kind of been on the back burner. I think I can really only handle one monumental crisis at a time, and you know, at this point, we're kind of crossing our fingers, because there's just not a whole lot to do at the moment."

"Well, that's good," he said. "I'm happy to hear that."

We did receive the official diagnosis after my trip to the ER with my dad. My dad's general practitioner told my mom he was sorry, that he wouldn't wish this on anyone. As my dad was still, at that point, the primary breadwinner for my parents and his earning potential had just been clipped in a matter of moments, the next year plus was a logistical whirlwind for them: shutting down my dad's practice, moving.

But since that time, things had been manageable; there had been a reprieve for everyone involved. He was there. He might have difficulty finding the exact right word he was looking for when telling a story, but it was a rare occasion when I couldn't figure out pretty quickly what he was talking about. That ebbed and flowed a little bit, but the doctor said he had been astonished, and that many did not get this chance. To hold it at bay, even for a little while, was no small feat.

He said, inevitably though, things were going to change.

I think part of my reactions to the deaths of my friend David and my Uncle Bill was some sort of dissatisfaction with how fast they happened—the deaths and the aftermaths. A moment of shocking news, a few months of craziness, and then they were gone, and it seemed there really wasn't a whole lot more to say about it. And I, for one, felt as if I needed more time to sum things up.

Well, the alternative, obviously, is not any better—dragging the death out in a horrible way for many years. I suppose, in a way, it has given me more time to think about what to say, about how to possibly memorialize a life, or how to eulogize my father. In retrospect, though, that's not actually what I had in mind. But I have gone through this mental exercise of eulogy-writing a bit recently, not really by choice.

At my older sister's rehearsal dinner roughly a decade ago, my father's speech quoted from "When I'm Sixty-Four,"[80] one of his favorite songs. I first thought that at his eventual eulogy if I really wanted to make people cry or, at the least, make myself cry (if that is the point of a eulogy), I could just read "When I'm Sixty-Four" in its entirety. That would probably be sufficient. I could maybe simultaneously play the air banjo, or else the air maracas.

Then again, maybe I could use his own words. I found a letter my dad

---

[80] The Beatles, "When I'm Sixty-Four" (Parlophone, 1967).

had sent me in conjunction with a Catholic weekend retreat that I attended in high school. The letter read, in part:

> I remember the days when you were three or four years old when you would come in at night to my side of the bed, and I would pull you up into bed with us…We are all constantly learning new things in our existence and new ways of coping with life…always use your common sense and your conscience, and you will be fine.

Coping, unfortunately, is right. Some things cannot be traded away; some times can only be coped with.

At my dad's mom's funeral, though, the sentiment was more positive. My dad read *Love You, Forever*, the children's book,[81] in its entirety. My little sister was still a baby at the time, so the book was floating around, and my parents were very fond of it. I was ten or eleven. The mother cares for her son throughout his life and sings a refrain after he goes to bed: "I love you forever, I like you for always, as long as I'm living, my baby you'll be." In the end, the son sings the same refrain to his own mother, when she is old and in need of help, and then, to his own kids. I was told recently that this book is actually divisive, and a lot of people think it's creepy. Maybe it is; I don't know. I haven't reviewed the critical analysis of *Love You Forever* recently. But, in the end, it might be too openly heartfelt for me.

Or finally, another option: during one break in my semester in Nottingham, in May 2002, my friend Peter and I spent a week walking in the Peak District in England. We'd hike through fields and valleys during the day and stay in B&Bs and visit small town pubs at night. During one of our days in Derbyshire, we passed through an English country church and cemetery, Edensor Chapel. One tombstone epitaph caught my eye and inspired me to scratch it down:

> "Not now but in the coming years, it may be in the better land, we'll read the meaning of our tears and then sometime we'll understand. Henry Joseph Smedley, born July 7, 1864, fell asleep November 11, 1914."

I think this is the quote that works best for me. I may not now "understand" many things that happen: fast-spreading, spontaneous cancer

---

[81] Robert Munsch, *Love You Forever* (Firefly Books, 1986).

that can fell a man in months, mind-blowing and heartless dementia, a misstep and a fall. There is hope, though, that sometime, perhaps later in life or, you know, elsewhere—because it appears that hoping for some sort of adequate summing up here seems unlikely—we'll gain wisdom. Not comfort necessarily, but understanding, because understanding would be nice. Having those times make sense would be nice. Having it all matter, of course, would also be nice.

***

I think "fertility trail" is probably wrong. Unless we're talking about some sort of Overlook Trail, the Phelps Lake Trail,[82] the path named for its end destination. More accurately, this experience was the Road *to* or the Trail *to* Fertility. I long for there to be a Fertility, Tennessee, somewhere, a countryside Xanadu, that we could visit and take a few Instagram photos of ourselves: "FERTILITY, TENNESSEE. Population: You two bad asses." You made it. You have arrived. You are fertile. You are pregnant.

Because going the way we were going, it was not as if we were gradually becoming more fertile as we stumbled along. Bountiful plants and bunches of bounding animals, freed from a robot curse,[83] were not suddenly bouncing around us on all sides having multiplied in gross as we passed by and exuded a sense of our fecund essence. Arguably, of course, the laparoscopy made us more fertile, but you're going to have a tough time convincing any decent judge of that argument. No, the process is a "to." A Trail to Fertility, where we seemed forever lost in the process, the journey, the infertility.

***

We decided to move forward with the frozen transfer immediately. At that point, it seemed fairly obvious. The embryos were there, revved up and waiting to go, which meant no retrieval. The transfer itself would only cost about $2,000, which—relatively speaking—was cheap. We would have to buy more drugs, but not as many as before because there would be no need for follicle stimulation. Obviously, continuing the same course wasn't ideal, but we still had confidence in our doctor, and our doctor still had confidence that he could make this happen. Plus, at the very least, we needed to take advantage of the fact that we had been able to produce so many viable embryos. We had

---

[82] See Grand Teton National Park.
[83] See *Sonic the Hedgehog* (Sega, 1991).

lucked out there and maybe nowhere else at any point during this process, so we needed to take advantage of that luck.

The DD said we didn't need to wait any specific amount of time, which we were happy to hear, as waiting at this point seemed fundamentally out of the question. So we started the process almost immediately. On March 13, my wife began taking birth control pills again with a goal for a transfer around the end of April. [End of March drugs: $45.90 + $130.34.]

We decided, for this trip, that we were going to get a hotel room. First and foremost, it is worth making a special mention of the support we had from Q. and her husband and family during the first transfer. I'm not sure how it would have worked in Dallas otherwise. My wife flew in on February 10 and stayed for two full weeks, and the hospitality was perfect, exceedingly generous. Q. was always game for injecting Julie with whatever medicine was needed, always willing to hear all about how the process works and the entire ridiculous experience, and she never made Julie feel that any of it was a burden in any way. My wife was upset when leaving, in part, because the entire thing had been such a positive, bonding experience.

For this one, it made far more sense to get a hotel room (using hotel points) and simply hang out together in Dallas for four days. The three-week thing was different: It would not have been feasible if Julie couldn't have stayed with Q. Here, this was only going to be a few days. It was time to make the process entirely about the two of us and our family. No one else was going to be involved, and that's how it should have been.

Plus, at the time, we understandably were "raw" emotionally: raw, turkey carcasses with tiny, little, T-Rex arms. Likewise, we had blinders on, deep on the Trail to Fertility, which at this point, was completely overgrown around us, blocking out the sunlight and our connection with the rest of the world, with no markers, no path, nothing in sight, other than this one option, this next step, this one bare foot forward. Thus, we felt a certain amount of distance from other people, who were not as lost and confused as we were.

I do think this distance is an inevitable outgrowth of this process, something you may certainly encounter deep on the Trail. In the end, there is simply something about this entire experience that separates you from others. Unless the other person has actually been through it, I think it's difficult for these outsiders to know how to possibly communicate with you. As such, at this point, it just didn't make sense to stay with friends and explain or even discuss the matter any more. We were on our own.

One of my wife's friends told her, while we were in the middle of all of this, that she just didn't know what to say. I think she was right.

***

The frozen cycle was anticipated to be much less burdensome. Julie did have to take the Lupron shots (smaller, in the stomach) again so that the doctors could control/prevent ovulation. She took these for about four weeks, and halfway through, my wife tacked on the estrogen patches and progesterone shots. So, for two weeks leading up to the transfer, we were again engaging in two progesterone shots per day. We had had a month off, but they were back. At this point, we had learned to heat the syringe full of liquid, wrapped in a heating pad, for five or ten minutes before entry. Then we would ice down the backside with a leaky Ziploc of frozen-and-re-frozen ice cubes, but otherwise it was the same: a honking needle, a bare backside, avoiding bruises, searching for clean entry.

Julie had an intralipid infusion at a Walgreens the Monday before we left. [$78.18.] On Thursday evening, April 26, we flew to Dallas. [$226.10 times two + $129 for drugs around this time + $325 times two for two trips to the TFC before we left for ultrasounds.]

We rented a car and proceeded to our Sheraton "suite" complete with small refrigerator—and microwave! Our hotel window looked out over a Medieval Times right next door. I thought this hilarious, because it was. The next morning we got up early, went to the wondrous Central Market, and wandered its bounteous halls, seizing on fresh tortillas and fresh-squeezed orange juice, fresh breakfast tacos and coffee (for me).

My wife had made appointments with an acupuncturist for both before and a few days after the transfer. My cousin, who lives in Dallas, had recommended a particular doctor. The idea was to do all we could to ease the nerves and calm anxiety before the actual transfer. Thus, after Central Market, we traveled through Dallas's construction-stunted roads scouring for office parks. We discovered the acupuncturists, a Chinese physician man and wife, in a brick building immediately off of a primary thoroughfare. The doors to their office were hidden in a little enclave pouch in the middle of the building. I sat in the waiting room and tried to read sports articles on my phone. The office was busy, and the clientele were definitely women in their twenties and thirties. The acupuncturists gave us more advice: Alkaline foods were good; acidic foods were bad. In other words we should eat plenty of kiwi and beets, not as much lamb and ice cream. [$75.]

It was clear to me that, on this particular trip, perhaps more so than others, a positive attitude was vitally necessary. I understood that Julie worried and I was well aware that during the last procedure, the transfer itself and the bed rest had not been a stress-less experience. Thus, throughout this trip, I was—against my nature—attempting to have a fully positive, blissfully unaware, highly consciously uncritical take on the matter. I bought into this approach, so it wasn't as if I was secretly sniveling at everything the DD said, as I appear to be doing now. No, I was happy. In fact this trip, in my memory, was an extremely positive one. We essentially had a hotel vacation with nothing external to worry about; in fact, the only goal of the trip was not to worry period, about anything.

***

On the morning of the transfer itself, at the DD's office, the DD's wife (the office manager) made a passing comment that my wife needed to stay calm, to be more relaxed, less anxious. I noted it at the time, even in my trusting state, because it appeared that was probably their excuse behind closed doors: She's too anxious. That troubled me.

Because was that the secret diagnosis? Would that mean she was too anxious to ever undergo this process? Or too anxious to ever get pregnant? Must a pregnancy occur by sleight of hand? Isn't everyone anxious through an IVF transfer? By definition, if you find yourself at this stage, there's a problem. And if there is some type of "problem" with a couple's ability to make a baby, and they clearly want one, then I anticipate some type of anxiety. In the end, after the revolving door of various maladies, is their expert opinion that she's just an anxious person, and that's why it didn't work?

We were led through the double doors into the second half of the office, the hospital, Dr. Jekyll side—Mr. Hyde and his porn collection stay on the other—and deposited into the room we had been assigned to before, still cold. The wait was nothing notable, and the preparation was nothing much. My wife was given a Valium before we were led across the hall to the operating room. I was invited this time.

They wheeled Julie in and positioned her hospital bed headboard against one wall. A stool was provided near her head for me to perch on and keep her company. I was called over, however, by the embryologist—the embryo maker. He beckoned me to one corner of the room where there was a scientific contraption, like in infectious disease movies, a microscope, and a place to put both hands through large gloves to handle the organism inside. He told me to go ahead and take a look. I looked where I was told and saw the microscopic image of what were apparently the two embryos: round bundles that looked like they were about to start growing like Gremlins in water, cells spontaneously replicating, bursting off the backs of others.[84]

The embryologist clearly wanted me to be impressed by the process, by the embryos, by what were apparently the results of his hard, painstaking work, and by what was about to happen. And from far away, perhaps I can marvel at what wonders can be accomplished by man. But at the time, I thought this, frankly, was not the hospital nursery. I was stilted, awkward probably; I nodded and retreated to my wife's side.

The process was exceedingly brief. Along with the embryologist, the DD was there with two or three nurses. The embryos I had seen were extracted from their chamber and injected directly into the uterus. I held my wife's hand tight for about twenty seconds when the syringe went in, but it was over quickly. In moments, we were back in our original room, where my wife received another intralipid transfer. Orangish, yellow fat in the IV bag, into her arm.

Julie was supposed to lie still in the hospital room for a couple of hours at least; it seemed like more. We thought our nurse had forgotten us. She had not. I think I may have paid for something at that point. Swiped the credit card. [$2,123.] Eventually, our nurse allowed us to go. She helped me wheel my wife to the elevator and to the downstairs parking garage and our car. The elevator stopped on the main floor, and the smell of popcorn permeated.

We were left alone to maneuver the construction that wrapped us in a square, all four corners, around the building, right, right, right, and left before we had to manage the interstate tangle of bomb wires in order to make it back to our Medieval Times overlook. At one point on this relatively short trip, I knew I had to get into the right lane in order to make our way to the appropriate exit off the interstate, but I had not made an attempt soon enough and was forced at the last moment to jerk over and force my way in to a long line of cars with a momentary jabbing of brakes. That was obviously not something I could worry about at the time and, in the end, not even something I could worry about after the time. Because if that little variable could have had any real, discernible effect on this process, then it was simply not worth the money, the discomfort, or the emotional renting, and those who perform it should force the patients to be locked in an underground bunker at the hospital so that every aspect of this delicate process could be managed. Or, maybe, a four-day, drug-induced coma. It couldn't possibly have had an effect…

She remained on bed rest through the weekend. Our hotel party was

---

[84] See *Gremlins* (Warner Bros., 1984).

great—remarkably stress-free. I would pop out each day back to Central Market or another high-end Dallas, prepared-food store to pick out easily reheatable dinners. I taught her how to play chess. We watched *Ratatouille*.[85] I called my friend Peter who lived in Fort Worth to see if he would go to Medieval Times with me. (He was out of town.) We watched *Contagion*;[86] we watched the worst movie in the history of the world, *Helena from the Wedding*.[87] We ate tortillas and sometimes heavily alkaline food, like sweet potatoes. I drank beer. On the final day, we took an adventure to the swimming pool and read books.

On Monday, April 30, after our trip to the pool, my wife had another acupuncture treatment, same doctor, just an entirely different office nowhere near the other. This one was way out in the flat, Texas landscape off a brand new highway to what seemed like nowhere, in nowhere. Frisco? We drove down memorial highways that looked like they should have ramps as cars sped by at high rates. I was more careful this time, though, with no traffic scares. The acupuncturist, even in this seemingly frontier establishment, was crowded as usual, with more women in their twenties and thirties. [$105 this time, for some reason.] We flew home Tuesday morning, May 1. [Rental car: $220.60; Fly Away parking in Nashville: $46.67; Texas tolls: $13.93.]

***

The first pregnancy test was planned for the following Monday, May 7, 2012, at OB2's office. We casually went back to work and through a normal weekend, ignoring the obvious.

That Monday, my wife went in and took a blood test. I was not exactly sure when the call would come. The last time, it seemed the calls came with no discernible pattern—sometimes late in the afternoon, sometimes early in the afternoon, or at one point, near the end of the day. A co-worker sent out an e-mail asking the other associates in my firm to lunch. I thought going about my day as I normally would was the proper course of action. Sitting in my office worrying, changing customary decision-making based on the fact that I may receive news at any point in time, seemed like the wrong way to approach it. Maintain hope, but at the same time, maintain normalcy.

Which meant I went with the group across West End to a spot that now

---

[85] *Ratatouille* (Disney, 2007).

[86] *Contagion* (Warner Bros., 2011).

[87] *Helena from the Wedding* (Beech Hill Films, 2010).

no longer exists, called Pie in the Sky Pizza. I had gone there a few times and never had actually ordered the pizza, which was a mistake. Going was also probably a mistake. In hindsight, I should have just holed up in my office, shut the door, eaten a burrito, and stared at the phone. Then again, the concern about what I should have done in hindsight ceases to have any meaning for me. In the end, it did not matter one way or the other what I did or what I happened to be doing at the time.

Sure, if I was scarfing down a pepperoni calzone or buffalo chicken sandwich, my ability to comfort my wife via the telephone might be impeded in a significant capacity, but depending on what the news was going to be, my instant ability to comfort seemed to be drained of importance. They would be meaningless, empty, mechanical words, because she would know that I felt the same way she did. Anything I would say would dissolve into bromides, maybe another "We'll get through this." No shit. We will get through this, just by existing. If there was a high chance, a distinct possibility, that emotional moments and/or massive disappointment might cause someone to spontaneously combust into flame, burn away, and die, perhaps we should congratulate ourselves for getting through something like this, suffering through something like this. But, under these circumstances, it appeared to me that the only way you "got through" this, such that you could look back and say, "Wow, we really got through that," is if you had a baby in tow on the other end. Then, yeah, you "got through it."

Of course, my phone started buzzing while I was sitting in the pizza shop. I nonchalantly scampered out of the door of the place and onto a sidewalk. Negative pregnancy test. It did not work.

The news was a physical sensation, a wave through my body, radiating from the head and moving down. Then I found that it had passed, gone through, and I was quickly back in normalcy. This normalcy just had a slant to it, a depressing, slanted roof that swung into place overhead, well-constructed, strongly supported, and there.

I expressed disappointment. I said I was sorry. I said I'd call her back in ten minutes. I knew Julie would probably call her parents or sister anyway—not that I was outsourcing comforting responsibility, because I wasn't. I knew Julie didn't think that, but I'm sure she knew that I was simply incapable of telling her much right then that would help. Maybe some sort of objective third-party might be able to say positive things, although I doubted it. But I knew whatever I said would not be positive. Then again, did we even need positivity at this point? Need to discuss the future? Next steps? I would have preferred to be there to provide physical comfort, but there was nothing to talk about.

Later that week, Friday maybe, we were trying to see a movie. Even though we live only two miles from the movie theater, we somehow managed to start screaming at each other before we got there, and I was so angry that I U-turned it and went home. What the conflicting positions were I don't remember, but I remember I was angry because someone had mentioned surrogacy recently, just casually to us, perhaps not entirely seriously, I don't know. I don't think Julie was actually bringing it up to discuss as a real possibility because she was obviously as burned out as I was, but the mere mention of the word riled me, made me want to splatter about, and I said something along the lines of "I don't want to talk about fucking surrogacy." I didn't want to talk about it, think about it, contemplate it, or say it. I felt the reasons were fairly obvious, but if I needed to list them, I could. The first and far most important, pivotal reason that existed—and actually, on second thought, I don't think I need to delve into any others, one was good enough—was that I AM NOT A MOVIE STAR. I'm not.

***

After the negative pregnancy test, Julie did get to peel off the estrogen patches. She stopped taking the progesterone shots. No more needles twice a day, every day. We got to stop.

We had a call with the DD that Saturday. We took no notes. He mentioned that there could be an issue with the "quality" of my wife's eggs, something he had flatly denied in our call after the first failed cycle, when he said the slow growth did not matter, that all embryos were different, and that it did not indicate anything. This time, he said the slow growth could have been indicative of a problem. He had gone to a conference last weekend, where there had been an interesting paper presented that discussed this possibility, or probability.

His old-man mannerisms were less apparent and his wandering, distant tone that we had determined was charming, I guess, was not there. He made his points normally, with no attempt at comfort or consolation. There seemed, in his voice, a tinge of annoyance. My quick calculus was that we were having a negative effect on his success rates. He was at a loss as to why, but he had too many other patients that were equally paying and were not as adverse to success. This simply was not good for him. Or, if I'm being fair, maybe this was just the worst part of his job.

I, on the other hand, was dumbfounded. Went to a conference? I understood our treatment was fairly "cutting-edge," but goodness, I did not know it was something that changed conference-to-conference, weekend in Palm Beach to weekend in Palm Beach. I was unaware that he, a supposed expert with success rates significantly higher than anyone else in the country, was learning something new at every conference he went to, so things he may tell us one week would become patently untrue the next. It now seemed that he didn't know what he was doing any more than the woman at the TFC: point and shoot. It had been twenty months and we still were not even able to trust this natural killer cell hypothesis or otherwise explain why we were incapable of getting pregnant—we still did not even have a diagnosis! Egg quality? Fuck that.

In the end, my dissatisfaction with the bedside manner of certain physicians is clear. Maybe we were not paying for that, and maybe we were paying for expertise (or actually results, as this is a results-oriented business). If that was the case, though, why did we ever bother meeting doctors at all? Let them come in via a secret, glass suction tube, do what they needed to do, and then leave. Instead, they should just designate a nurse, who has a clue as to the doctor's decision-making and thoughts, who could be there for both nurse services and comfort. We had a nurse who didn't know what was going on, and then a doctor who was guilted into periodically having phone calls with his patients, where he pulls back the curtain and lets you know that, well, really, he had no idea, either.

I don't think kind, comforting words were necessary to convince us that things were going to get better, or it was eventually going to work out, or that they had any other logical benefit. But, in the end, I would say they do help to make the patient feel that this entire endeavor was not a sham and that it was not a complete waste of money, emotional stability, and enormous, hand-ripped, rotisserie chicken meat chunks of time.

Somewhere in California

"Tamandua!"

If I'm trying to articulate meaning—what my father taught me, what a son learned from a father[88]—there is certainly something here. The old refrain from my youth was that if I got a bad grade, I should tell my mom, and if I got into any trouble, I should tell my dad. Bad grades weren't necessarily an issue, but I certainly got into plenty of trouble. It was true that it was preferable to first tell my father. Doing so would not necessarily abate the gathering storm of my mother, who tended to have more emotional, initial reactions to unfavorable news, but my father was a mild-mannered, thoughtful, rational person, or, as Julie has said, a "sweet man." And it made more sense to broach the news with him first and hope that a little bit of that reason would transfer to my mother before she decided to make her feelings known.

One such problem I got myself into was different, though, and marked the one and only time I can remember that my father truly got angry with me—furious, in fact. The one time my dad out-tiraded my mom.

The summer after my sophomore year in high school, I went on a school-sponsored trip to Italy and Greece. The trip was amazing, but I was sixteen and stupid. On the last night of the trip, I decided it would be seriously awesome if I partied all night until it was time to leave for the plane ride home at 5:00 a.m.; instead, I crashed and barfed on the streets of Athens in front of my

---

[88] Another potential book title: *Catawampus: A Random Thirty-Something Male's Journey from Boy or, You Know, Young Adult Still Trailing the Streams of the Juvenile to Man or Adult, I Guess, While Trying to Become a Father While in the Process He Happened to be Losing His Own Father and Such.*

future Latin IV: *Aeneid*[89] teacher before dinner.

Later that summer, I had to appear before my school's disciplinary council, ten of the most intimidating and well-respected teachers at the school, sitting around a small table staring at me and giving me a hard time. I, in turn, stared at the edge of the table and avoided eye contact. Needless to say, they took me down a notch. After the meeting, my parents asked me what I told the council when they asked if I had been drinking alone that fateful evening. I told them what I had said, that I had been solo. My dad was very angry.

It was clear to everyone associated with the situation that I had lied; I roomed with two friends of mine that night, and the idea that I would be slamming drinks in a corner while the two of them looked on in fascination was fairly preposterous. As a sixteen-year-old, though, certain value systems were far more important to me than pure honesty. One of my high school's most famous alumni was Sam Davis, a Confederate spy, caught and executed by Union troops, who was purported to have said that he would rather die a thousand deaths than betray a friend. What did everyone think I was going to do? At the time, it sounded noble to me to fall on my sword for my friends, and of course, it was clearly my own fault that this trouble occurred in the first place. I assumed the teachers at my school were at least partly aware of why I did what I did, although that might have been a tad naïve. I did not, however, anticipate my father's reaction.

He said no matter what, I should not have lied. He never told me that I should have ratted out my friends, but he did say I should not have lied. I tried to explain the situation, that he just did not understand, that I couldn't tell the truth, but he was not interested. He brushed the explanations aside and said that the matter was simple: I should never have lied.

So if we're looking for something tangible, this is what a father taught his child: the supreme importance of honesty. Always.

Otherwise, father as hero is an old trope, but even with my dad, I've got a story. When I was around four or five, strapped into a car seat with my older brother and sister in the back with me, the happy family of five in a Volkswagen Rabbit was coming out of the old Baskin-Robbins in Belle Meade, where West End (now Harding Road) splits into Highway 100 and Highway 70, both of which race off in the direction of Bellevue and far West Nashville.

I imagine we had been to Shoney's for dinner earlier that evening before stopping for dessert. When the light turned green, the Rabbit scampered into the awkward intersection and immediately got run over by a drunk driver;

---

[89] See Virgil, *The Aeneid* (19 B.C.).

scoops of mint chocolate chip slowly twirling through the air. The story I learned later, as I have no memory of any of this (other than waking up naked on a table, being examined by aliens), is that my father stuck his arm in front of my mother who was in the passenger seat. His forearm took the impact that my mother's chest would have otherwise. His arm snapped, but otherwise, no one was seriously injured.

We grew up for the first thirteen years of my life on a twenty-three-acre farm in Bellevue. Over the years, we had horses, chickens, rabbits, turkeys, peacocks—I think a cow or two before I was born. One evening my dad's cousin's wife, who was, in general, apparently a hysterical person, came over with a dead cat in a box and insisted my dad bury it for her on our property. We had buried our old Great Dane, Rommel, down by one of our lakes, but it was not as if we were operating a pet cemetery. At the time, it was the dead of winter and my father and one of my other maternal uncles, who was living in a detached apartment on the property at the time, hiked down to the lake and tried to finagle a hole out of the earth. But it was freezing and the earth wasn't budging. After a while, it seemed like a hopeless endeavor, and you know, well, what was the difference? They tossed the box into the trashcan and went back inside. Another story I heard growing up definitely seems to not be entirely true, but is something that has grown in familial legend over time. One day, my father allegedly came into the house and told my older sister that her rabbit, Homer, was outside in the front yard. Technically, only part of Homer was. The other half we later found in the loft of the barn, transported by owl, we presumed. I cannot imagine this story is in fact, true, as it is a bit callous, but it's morphed into great family lore, and, for some reason, both of these dead animal stories have always made me laugh.

So, my dad was a skeptic perhaps, or, else, a practical man, who, needless to say, knew the pleasure of a good, solid joke.

My father worked for more than forty years, day-in and day-out. I cannot remember his missing a day. I cannot remember his complaining about his day. He was simply always up, always waking us up for school by turning off our fans, always driving us to school, and always there at dinner at night. He was forced to retire abruptly after his diagnosis. The building was sold, his practice was turned over to his partner, and most of the owl paintings were left behind. The practice eventually teamed up with a chain—what appeared to be a self-proclaimed, famous ophthalmologist, who slapped his name on the building and maybe periodically made an appearance—but that was almost two years after my father had gone.[90] My parents were not terribly social people, and all the rest of us were simply afraid, to be honest, after the diagnosis and in no mood for celebrating. So we never even had a basic retirement party—never even went to dinner to celebrate forty years of hard work, my father's life's work.

It was tragic in a way…although maybe not. The Joseph Conrad quote, for some reason, comes to mind: "I don't like work—no man does—but I like what is in the work —the chance to find yourself. Your own reality—for yourself not for others—what no other man can ever know. They can only see the mere show, and never can tell what it really means."[91] How's this: My father exemplified this concept. He didn't care. He hadn't worked all of his life for a fist-bump party at the end.

There were a few events later in life, before the diagnosis, where in hindsight, it was tough to determine whether it was simply my dad being my dad, Terry being Terry, or whether the disease might have been manifesting itself a little bit. One was at a Predators' game, where the corrupt NHL referees had, once again, caused the team to lose. We had seats on the railing over the referees' exit ramp and somehow—my dad claimed accidentally—his cup of water went catapulting over the side and landed squarely in a referee's face as he was leaving the ice. I think that was probably more than likely my dad being my dad, and you know, those motherfuckers deserved it. Another lesson learned: Fight corruption in all its forms, any way you know how.

Another time, my little sister had been out on Old Hickory Lake[92] all day with her friends. At some point she had decided to ditch two jet-skis that my parents owned by simply tying them to a tree in the water. I think she figured they could just get it the following day. Somehow this got communicated to my parents at 10:00 or 10:30 p.m., and they informed her that was not acceptable, because, hey, free jet-ski.[93]

This meant my sixty-plus-year-old parents raced out to the lake, and the three of them went onto the water at midnight to retrieve the crafts. My mom

---

[90] For what it's worth, Julie did stop by this office for one brief moment to pick up contacts a year or so later, and in the short stretch of time she was there, she overheard an elderly patient asking the woman at the front desk about Dr. B. The desk clerk indicated that Julie was his daughter-in-law. The woman accosted Julie, told her what a great doctor my father had been to her, and how she wished he was still there.

[91] See Joseph Conrad, *Heart of Darkness* (Blackwood's Magazine, 1899).

[92] Old Hickory was Andrew Jackson's nickname. His home, The Hermitage, is just east of Nashville.

[93] See Jack Handey, *Deep Thoughts* (Berkley Trade, 1992) ("Hey, free dummy.").

drove the boat, and, on the way back, my dad and little sister drove the two jet-skis. They were supposed to follow close behind because the jet-skis didn't have lights, and it was pitch black on the water.

At one point on the journey, though, a barge came around the bend, because Old Hickory Lake is also the Cumberland River—the river that winds its way from northeast Davidson County to downtown Nashville. My mother assumed she didn't need to tell my dad that he should stay out of the way and wait it out. He had other plans though and, for some reason, went speeding across the water directly in the path of the onrushing barge. I cannot imagine what the driver must have thought to see this mustachioed sixty-four-year-old jumping waves in front of a barge at midnight in sheer darkness. (I'm thinking for the *Catawampus* movie, Wayne Coyne[94]—or maybe Beaker[95]—can play Mr. Barge Driver. "What is this?" before my dad goes flying over a wave, slow motion through the air, with jet-ski motor humming.) One final lesson learned: barge-dodging, try it.

So yeah, honestly, saving my mother and non-existent little sister's lives, dead cat in a trashcan, hard work, fighting corruption, barge-dodging? That's a pretty good legacy in my book. I hope I can do as much.

***

I have one final maternal uncle. This one lived in Brazil for a good part of his adult life. Our fourth year in college, Julie and I went to visit him over winter break, as he was planning an eventual move with his family back to the states, and this opportunity would not arise again.

At one point during the trip, he flew us into the interior wetlands, the Pantanal, for several days of outdoor activities. On our last outing, we hiked through a forest, body-floated down a river, and saw various wild beasts: We swam in a pool where sun-bathing alligators were collapsed half in the water, a meandering rodent the size of a basset hound passed us nonchalantly on the forest trail, and a toucan with its beak leading the way streaked over the trees. At the end of the day, on our bus ride back to Campo Grande, the bus driver pulled off to the side of the road and stopped. He got out and pointed to a neighboring field. "Tamandua!" he shouted. We waited our turn and tumbled off the bus.

A tamandua is a giant anteater, and one was galloping across empty

---

[94] Lead singer of The Flaming Lips.
[95] Orange-haired muppet.

farmland with the tuft of fur on its arching back flopping from side to side in the air.

On the morning of our wedding day, five or so years later, the *Washington Post* printed a large picture on the front page of a baby giant anteater, hanging onto its mama, apparently the first giant anteater born at the National Zoo. There had been some minor, stress-related tension between Julie and me the day before, so I tore out the picture, wrote "Tamandua!" on top, and slid it under her door.

Spotting that tamandua in Brazil might not have been important, but with time, I say that it was. And I like to think, at this point, as we were deep and lost on the Trail to Fertility, that in the trees, I might have noticed something out of the corner of my eye, a flash of the tamandua mohawk, or else, a quick glimpse of a big bushy tail before it scurried out of sight.

***

Obviously, we needed a break.

Whatever was happening had to stop. There would be no fertility treatments whatsoever and no plans for continued fertility treatments. We would stop everything, immediately. Beyond that, I don't think we had any idea, but for what seemed like the first time in a long time, the correct and only answer, no doubt whatsoever, was right in front of us: stop.

We had a friend who had trouble getting pregnant as well, but never went down or seemingly ever even considered the Western medicine route. (As one person said to me, "The *Western* route? As opposed to what?") She was from Texas and knew a woman, L., a homeopath (a health nut of sorts) in California. She had contacted L. for assistance and, after years of not having a period at all, she got her period after two months of L.'s "remedies." These remedies consisted of "homeopathics," i.e., herbal supplements, like say, Crab Apple Bud, pills of salt-like minerals with rock-like descriptions of their ingredients (zirconium, for instance) that you let dissolve on your tongue and liquids in little vials we later called "potions" that our "witch-doctor" had sent us. Four months after our friend's period resumed, she was pregnant.

Obviously, the story was an incredible one. I remember hearing it at the time and considering it a good story but, clearly, I thought, she was different from us. We had a "problem" that had been plaguing us from the beginning and for twenty months since. We had an issue that desperately needed scientific or medical fixing or bypassing or Froggering[96] over and, I don't know, perhaps our friend just couldn't get her period for a while.

At the same time, it seemed worthwhile to give this a shot. We were going to be taking a break from all other types of treatment and, unlike everything else we had been doing to my wife's body, to our time, bank accounts, and emotional health, this would not be hurting anything. While we took a break, we could try some all-natural remedies, just for laughs, so that we could feel like we were still doing something. And, simultaneously, we could take a break and get back to just good old-fashioned "trying." Julie was also planning on continuing with acupuncture and, at this point, started seeing her acupuncturist weekly.

My wife e-mailed L. on May 8, 2012 and scheduled a call with her on May 15. (She got her period on May 10.) L.'s theory was that years on the Pill, plus all of the exogenous hormones my wife had put into her body with the IVF cycles had clogged her system. She said a month of her remedies eliminated a year's worth of toxins, but that this was a process and would take time. Julie had been on the Pill for eight years and then off of it for about two and a half years at this point, so theoretically, we had a ways to go. L. sent my wife her "protocol," which was a barrage of these homeopathic remedies, and she began taking them on May 22. [Consultation: $125; homeopathics: $423.78.][97]

The minute the second IVF failed, Julie also changed her diet and eliminated gluten. She had read somewhere about links between gluten and infertility, plus gluten and thyroid disorders, and decided to try this on her own. Around that time, my mother-in-law referenced, in passing, that my wife had been allergic to wheat as a child, and apparently, at one point, the gluten caused a rash to break out on her face. Now Julie suspected, at the least, a possible intolerance after years of minor indigestion issues.

L. was less concerned with eliminating gluten entirely, but she told her to cut out everything but Ezekiel bread, to cut out dairy (except goat's milk), to eat only organic fruits and vegetables, no pork, and very little sugar. Organic wine was OK, dark beer was OK. She also had her take Epsom salt baths. Apparently these help eliminate toxins from the body and my wife started taking two to three a week.

L.'s first e-mail read, in part:

For the first month, we are detoxifying the hormones out of the tissues,

---

[96] Frogger (Sega/Gremlin, 1981).

[97] We had spent $27,835.20 (or thereabouts) before our contact with L.

rebuilding the good flora to eliminate the exogenous hormones, supporting the liver, regulating the neuro vegetative nervous system, and giving you Vitamin E and an anti-oxidant for fertility.

For the second month, we are working to regulate the function of the liver (which manufactures hormones) and regulating the hormonal system with the plant buds—the first two weeks, we are working to move stagnation and the following two weeks of the cycle, we are supporting the body to build progesterone. The gammadyn Cu is an important mineral that is bound out with medication and is needed to support the enzymatic systems, especially fertility.

I'd heard many explanations over the past two years and, like many others, this seemed to make sense—or actually, let me be clearer: the e-mail didn't make any sense at all. It was gibberish as far as I could tell, but the overall theory certainly seemed to have some merit. We had been artificially controlling the natural, biological menstrual cycle for years and years by pumping external hormones into the body. Perhaps a good all-natural cleansing is exactly what Julie needed.

Plus, it was not as if we were buying in wholeheartedly or that I had to fundamentally believe that everything she was saying was 100 percent true. An even greater blessing though was that I didn't have to consciously ignore anything, either: distracted doctors, absentee doctors, annoyed doctors, and the host of harried nurses in their wake. Likewise, I didn't have to buy into some new and creative medical problem that spontaneously appeared and had to be overcome with some new treatment. This was something different: Take some remedies, get the body healthy, don't worry about it.

And so it began. At this point in time, the idea was just to avoid obsessing over the whole thing for a change. Not, in a sense, be trying at all. We both, of course, semi-consciously knew to go ahead and "try" around the appropriate days, but it was definitely not something that was scheduled.

We went to a charity ball on June 10. (The end-of-the-party Krystal burgers were cold.) The week after, my wife had still not gotten her period.

Around Day Thirty-Six of her cycle, Julie called the DD's office to see if it was normal for it to take a while to get back onto a regular routine after an IVF cycle. They said it can, but to take a pregnancy test. Once it was determined it was negative, they would give her progesterone to help jump-start her period. As we were at that point, in the process of rebuilding good flora and/or believing a decent amount of what L. was telling us, we weren't about to start pumping artificial hormones back in. My wife mentioned this conversation with the DD to me and I was naturally reticent to have her take a pregnancy test, as it would obviously take us out of our newfound, suddenly carefree, free love, sundress-wearing lives.

And I can certainly see your point, June 2012 Stuart. There was no reason for it. If we, by some laughable circumstance, happened to be pregnant, then waiting a few more weeks would not matter. All that could come of taking a test was, I thought, more unnecessary heartache. We'd been, as I said, in a much better mindset—buying into L.'s tactics, thinking that, maybe we would stick with her a bit longer, for the foreseeable future actually. Maybe it made sense to think this way and realize that it might take time, months, to clean everything from the system and get a good fresh start. Worrying again about pregnancy tests and the like seemed a tad too soon for me.

Naturally, that Friday, June 15, Julie decided to go ahead and take a test. She went home that afternoon and urinated on a little plastic stick. She saw a faint double line. I got home after work, and she told me about it. As I remember it, I didn't think much. To me, it didn't necessarily mean anything. Faint lines were indications of nothing, and we weren't in a situation where we even should have been getting our hopes up in any capacity. We should have waited, I thought, but whatever. It was another non-answer. Another six maybe? Who knew where we were or where we should have been in our spiking HCG levels?

My wife called OB2's office. They told her to buy another brand, preferably the digital kind that either says PREGNANT or NOT PREGNANT, so we weren't trying to read lines, and to try it on Monday.

On Monday morning, Julie got up early and took a test. I cannot say that I particularly remember her getting up—maybe just in subconscious, stone-monster-shaping thought. When I actually realized that she was awake and out of bed though, it wasn't as startling as it should have been if I had been full-fledged and deep asleep. Julie had a look on her face that I could not place: blank in a positive way. I had just barely become aware of my surroundings. I was awake. Without speaking, she showed me the stick and it read...PREGNANT.

***

My wife went into OB2's office that Monday and had a blood test. It came back at seventy-four, higher, of course, than we had ever scored at any other time. At this point, Julie was off and running and, needless to say, I wasn't controlling my woman. She called the DD's office to ask about the intralipid treatment. She was understandably nervous that she might lose the pregnancy due to the abnormally high natural killer cell activity. The Dallas office was brusque and told her to "follow whatever orders our local practitioner recommended." Julie was upset because, as we all knew, OB2 wasn't familiar with the natural killer cell phenomenon. Julie then e-mailed L. and the acupuncturist. L. urged her not to have another infusion, said natural killer cell activity was something that occurred naturally and not to put any additional things into her body.

She wrote:

> Getting pregnant is a natural, biological function as are natural killer cells in early pregnancy. There are no studies that prove miscarriage if they are high. If this baby is meant to be, then it will be. Please do not mess with this. You got pregnant naturally, and we want to have a healthy baby. We do NOT want a sick baby due to medication.

The acupuncturist, likewise, said he could treat the natural killer cell activity with acupuncture. Our fertility trail guides had spoken.

OB2's office had Julie come in two days later to see if her levels were doubling. They came back at one seventy-five and her progesterone was thirty, very high. The doctor was pleased. Two weeks later she had some spotting, so she went in for an early ultrasound on July 2. Everything was fine—no heartbeat yet, but they said it was still too early to detect one, and the HCG levels were over twelve thousand! We went to St. Simons for the Fourth of July 2012, and my wife started spotting again at the end of the trip. She was vocally nervous, but I was not worried. Morning sickness and fatigue had begun at that point. We went in for another ultrasound the Monday we got back, and saw a bouncing bean and a heartbeat.

***

So there we were, collapsed on the dusty floor of the Trail or, like Alice,[98] sitting on a forest bench after the path has been brushed away, the forest itself has gradually disappeared around her, and she is left alone in one quiet space to weep. We were there, going nowhere with her, when a tree door cranked open to reveal a wonderful world of color beyond. Quickly, efficiently, and

---

[98] See *Alice in Wonderland* (Disney, 1951).

without our really even considering it, we were done. It was over.

I have no explanation. If we are applying Occam's Razor, perhaps anxiety is the simplest answer. But I'm still skeptical. If anxiety is the answer, when does that anxiety factor in? Is it just after embryo formation or else precisely when the embryos are right next to the uterus? Is it just on that day, that moment and only that moment, when we're not supposed to be anxious, we're not supposed to think about it?

Plus, how can it possibly be such a specific type of anxiety? My wife is a naturally anxious person, and she did not cease to be one before we had this success. If you specifically, consciously worry about getting pregnant does that somehow translate into a natural body reaction preventing pregnancy? But on the other hand, if you pretend that you're not worried about it, you can trick your body into making it happen? I don't know. If all of this ultra high-tech, baby-making technology hasn't quite figured out how to get around natural worrying, then we seem to be playing different sports: changing the nets on a basketball goal, while everyone's waiting on the soccer field.

I told Julie that L. could take all the credit she wanted. I'm fine and happy to say she did it, and I do not discount her, her methods, her theories, or anything else. As I mentioned before, this is a results-oriented business. I don't know if one month of her remedies had anything to do with it, and frankly, I don't care. Maybe she did do it. Either way, I am eternally grateful. I should send her flowers.

Or maybe it was karma somewhere that boomeranged back, maybe we had done enough penance.

Maybe it was the fact that around the time we got pregnant, I found an old coin from my childhood: an Indian head penny dated 1887. Many years ago, I had been at the Nashville Flea Market looking at coins with my dad. The coin-dealer had a large glass case with a hinged top that he would open to access the merchandise. At one point, while he was talking to my father, I put my hand in. I just wanted to touch something that looked interesting, and, unknowingly, the man shut the case and crushed my little finger. I don't remember what finger it was, and I don't remember the pain, but I do remember he gave me an Indian head penny in a plastic sleeve as recompense. I kept it ever since, somewhere stashed in old childhood drawers, childhood tins, childhood boxes, but I had not seen it in a long time. I had uncovered it recently at my parents' house, as they were in the process of moving. My father had not been doing well during the move. I pinned it to a corkboard over my computer at work.

Or maybe Julie did meet a guardian angel on an airplane. The story sounded somewhat strange at first in this modern day and age of constant bombardment with perversity, but right about this time, while traveling for work, my wife was seated next to a middle-aged man—older perhaps than that, retired. He struck up a conversation with her and intuitively seemed to know a significant amount about what had been going on in her life. He could see it in her face, perhaps, a physical toll. Maybe guessing the infertility wasn't so hard, although, that would seem like a pretty astute, pinpointed guess. He proceeded to speak to her about it. The conversation had a slight religious bent, but his ultimate message was that she would be successful. And unlike the multiple doctors we had passed through in our time, Julie felt like he knew what he was talking about when he said it. He then gave her a fifty-dollar bill. He told her to keep that money and, when our first baby was born, to buy the baby a gift. He gave her his address and told her to write him a note when that happened. Like I said, I was skeptical at first, as anyone would be, but I trust Julie. If she says it was genuine, then it was. And at this point, a guardian angel sounded about as good an explanation as any.

Fertility, Tennessee

"Do not cry, little baby."

I had a plan to include here a revolving slideshow of five thousand photos of my new, sweet, little baby girl coupled with all sorts of pleasurable anecdotes of our brief time with her. I would then end with a picture of myself, maybe wearing a turtleneck, giving a thumbs up, and a quote below the picture reading: "Be strong. Keep your head up. It'll all work out."

I jest, of course. But, yes, it was a dark and stormy night. I mean, literally, it was dark, because it was about 2:00 a.m., and it was pretty stormy. Tornado sirens wailed as a tornado moved through Davidson County in pursuit of Gallatin. We woke up because we thought my wife's mysterious bag of waters had broken (apparently, it had been by the barometric pressure, labor-inducing, donkey-headed sandman), but Julie wasn't sure. We debated whether to go to the hospital just yet.

The birthing class indicated we had twenty-four hours before we really needed to go in after the bag o' water's bursting, right? Or maybe I wasn't paying attention. No, I was; I even knew the answer "perineum" for our pin-the-tail-on-the-pregnant-woman segment, but I didn't say it because I was embarrassed. But we had scheduled car work to be done that morning at 7:00 a.m. I thought if we waited, we could swing by the hospital and see if it was a false alarm. If it was a false alarm, we could drop the car off and go to work. It would be far more efficient that way.

Then our power went out—a sign from on high that I was an idiot, perhaps. I finally woke up, and we proceeded to the hospital around 4:00

a.m., dodging trash cans[99] that had been catapulted onto the road in the wake of what was apparently a fairly minor tornado.

After that, I'll spare you the details, as this book is obviously about the journey, not the victory lap, not the sliding on my knees at the corner flag with my shirt covering my face, screaming to the heavens after pounding in the winning goal, a diving header, back post. And truly, I would rather not have this story end with me, standing with a shit-eating grin on my face, like a dog frolicking after a quarter horse on cobblestones, gobbling up hearty manure pellets, smug and satisfied, ranting on and on about the birth of my child! Oh, you wouldn't believe it! Amazing! A story that, although unique to each person, has been told and told better, many times before and will be told countless times, literally in the years to come.

Then again, this is the fun part: The intake nurses said we were lucky to come in when we did, because they had just moved all of the patients back into their rooms from the hallway once the tornado had finally screamed through. Had we heard it? They also said before even engaging in any tests that my wife's bag of waters had definitely broken.

"We could smell you when you walked in."

They said, as it was our first, we might not have the child until late that night or the next day. I knew better than to accept something some medical professional told me as gospel. Sure, I said, we'll see. Actually, of course, I was as sheep-like as ever. But they took us up to our room, we filled out paperwork, we met nurses who were about to go off shift. We got an epidural plugged in around seven o'clock when my wife was about five centimeters. (I think she had been through enough physical torment for this.) For the next five hours, we relaxed. I live-texted the whole affair to family members and Julie's close friends.

To cap things off, our labor nurse said she knew my father. She said my dad had operated on her daughter's eyes many years before when her daughter was eight. She said he had been a good doctor. Julie moved one centimeter an hour until around noon when OB2 arrived and said it was time to start pushing.

During the pushing process, OB2 mentioned that our daughter was a little "catawampus" in the birth canal. A little twisted, askew, pointed in the wrong direction. Catawampus. Not anything to be concerned about. She would figure it out. And she did. She righted herself and eventually came on out as a cone-headed, blue alien.

---

[99] More 8-bit Paperboy (NES, 1988) than Super Mario Kart (Super Nintendo, 1992).

I have few grand insights thus far, but I thought it remarkable when I looked at myself in the mirror a few weeks into the experience and saw my little baby, saw her mannerisms, her facial expressions.

And, then, a few weeks after that, we wrote her a little baby infant's book:

-Little baby smiles.
-Little baby thinks of her time in the lost ancient city of Mu and all she learned there.
-TAMANDUA!!! (Lots of tamanduas here, hanging out in Mu.)
-Little baby looks worried.
-Saber-toothed tigers chase little baby.
-They will not catch her. (Little baby and friends easily out-run tigers.)
-Little baby thinks.
-The Higgs Boson.
-Little baby cries.
-Why you cry, little baby?
-Why you cry?
-Do not cry, little baby.
-Do not cry.
-The sun is bright.
-The river is high. (Or, alternatively, "Da milk abounds."[100])
-And you are wearing a cute little suit with whales all over it.
-Do not cry, little baby.
-Do not cry.

(The tamanduas then slowly stroll away.)

---

[100] Actually, let's go with "Da milk abounds."

Acknowledgments

Clay Ezell, Peyton Bowman, Charlie Corts, Seth McInteer and Howell O'Rear of the McInteer & O'Rear law firm in Nashville; Megan Casey, Sarah Hargrove, Margie Quina, Susan Davis ("SpeciMEN" was her idea); my mother-in-law Linda Steadman, proprietor of Too Many Books in Roanoke, Virginia, who taught me about Mu and said that a baby infant, at times, looks like she is contemplating the theory of relativity (I said the theory of relativity was old news); Ann and Shad Steadman, Eileen Burkhalter Smith, my editor Carin Siegfried (I knew, almost immediately, that if the word "SNORT!" appeared in redline I probably needed to change something), and my mother and my father.

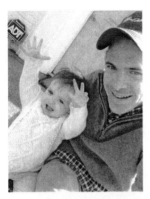

Stuart A. Burkhalter began writing creatively in college while studying abroad at the University of Nottingham in the spring of 2002. In 2003, his short story "Evidence of a Decision" won the Jefferson Literary and Debating Society's Annual Literary Contest at UVa. After college, he lived and worked in Washington, D.C. and New York City, and in his free time, wrote several short stories and screenplays. In 2005, Stuart and a friend produced *Of Age*, a 32-minute short film from one of Stuart's scripts. *Of Age* was accepted into multiple film festivals and, in 2006, won the Best Short Drama award at the Blue Ridge Mountain Southwest Virginia Vision Film Festival in Roanoke, Virginia. In 2007, he returned home to attend Vanderbilt University Law School. He graduated in 2010 and was elected a member of the Order of the Coif. In 2012, Stuart began writing what eventually became *Catawampus*.

Stuart is a graduate of the University of Virginia and Vanderbilt University Law School. He lives in Nashville with his family and is an attorney with Riley Warnock & Jacobson, PLC.

Visit Stuart at *www.stuartburkhalter.com*.